YO-EEV-926

Diabetes

Louise I. Gerdes, *Book Editor*

Daniel Leone, *President*
Bonnie Szumski, *Publisher*
Scott Barbour, *Managing Editor*

Contemporary Issues
Companion

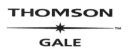

GREENHAVEN
PRESS ®

THOMSON
─────※─────™
GALE

San Diego • Detroit • New York • San Francisco • Cleveland
New Haven, Conn. • Waterville, Maine • London • Munich

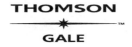

LIBRARY OF CONGRESS CATALOGING-IN-PUBLICATION DATA

Diabetes / by Louise I. Gerdes, book editor.
    p. cm. — (Contemporary issues companion)
Includes bibliographical references and index.
ISBN 0-7377-0838-7 (pbk. : alk. paper) — ISBN 0-7377-0839-5 (lib. : alk. paper)
    1. Diabetes. I. Gerdes, Louise I. II. Series.
RC660 .G47 2003
616.4'62—dc21   2002019386

Printed in the United States of America

CONTENTS

FOREWORD

In the news, on the streets, and in neighborhoods, individuals are confronted with a variety of social problems. Such problems may affect people directly: A young woman may struggle with depression, suspect a friend of having bulimia, or watch a loved one battle cancer. And even the issues that do not directly affect her private life—such as religious cults, domestic violence, or legalized gambling—still impact the larger society in which she lives. Discovering and analyzing the complexities of issues that encompass communal and societal realms as well as the world of personal experience is a valuable educational goal in the modern world.

Effectively addressing social problems requires familiarity with a constantly changing stream of data. Becoming well informed about today's controversies is an intricate process that often involves reading myriad primary and secondary sources, analyzing political debates, weighing various experts' opinions—even listening to first-hand accounts of those directly affected by the issue. For students and general observers, this can be a daunting task because of the sheer volume of information available in books, periodicals, on the evening news, and on the Internet. Researching the consequences of legalized gambling, for example, might entail sifting through congressional testimony on gambling's societal effects, examining private studies on Indian gaming, perusing numerous websites devoted to Internet betting, and reading essays written by lottery winners as well as interviews with recovering compulsive gamblers. Obtaining valuable information can be time-consuming—since it often requires researchers to pore over numerous documents and commentaries before discovering a source relevant to their particular investigation.

Greenhaven's Contemporary Issues Companion series seeks to assist this process of research by providing readers with useful and pertinent information about today's complex issues. Each volume in this anthology series focuses on a topic of current interest, presenting informative and thought-provoking selections written from a wide variety of viewpoints. The readings selected by the editors include such diverse sources as personal accounts and case studies, pertinent factual and statistical articles, and relevant commentaries and overviews. This diversity of sources and views, found in every Contemporary Issues Companion, offers readers a broad perspective in one convenient volume.

In addition, each title in the Contemporary Issues Companion series is designed especially for young adults. The selections included in every volume are chosen for their accessibility and are expertly edited in consideration of both the reading and comprehension levels of the audience. The structure of the anthologies also enhances accessibility. An introductory essay places each issue in context and provides helpful facts such as historical background or current statistics and legislation that pertain to the topic. The chapters that follow organize the material and focus on specific aspects of the book's topic. Every essay is introduced by a brief summary of its main points and biographical information about the author. These summaries aid in comprehension and can also serve to direct readers to material of immediate interest and need. Finally, a comprehensive index allows readers to efficiently scan and locate content.

The Contemporary Issues Companion series is an ideal launching point for research on a particular topic. Each anthology in the series is composed of readings taken from an extensive gamut of resources, including periodicals, newspapers, books, government documents, the publications of private and public organizations, and Internet websites. In these volumes, readers will find factual support suitable for use in reports, debates, speeches, and research papers. The anthologies also facilitate further research, featuring a book and periodical bibliography and a list of organizations to contact for additional information.

A perfect resource for both students and the general reader, Greenhaven's Contemporary Issues Companion series is sure to be a valued source of current, readable information on social problems that interest young adults. It is the editors' hope that readers will find the Contemporary Issues Companion series useful as a starting point to formulate their own opinions about and answers to the complex issues of the present day.

INTRODUCTION

Diabetes mellitus is a significant public health problem that affects about 17 million Americans, 6.2 percent of the population. While deaths due to cancer, stroke, and heart disease have declined since 1989, the death rates due to diabetes mellitus have increased by about 30 percent, and authorities estimate approximately 800,000 new cases will appear each year, increasing the number of Americans with diabetes to 23 million by 2010. Diabetes is the sixth leading cause of death in the United States. In 1999, diabetes resulted in more than 450,000 deaths, but many authorities believe this number is much greater because diabetes also contributes to deaths often attributed to other causes, including heart disease.

For those who have diabetes, the complications are what makes the disease so devastating. Diabetic retinopathy, an eye disease, is the leading cause of blindness in adults aged twenty through seventy-four. Diabetic nephropathy, a kidney disease, accounts for 40 percent of all new cases of end-stage renal disease, the final stage in a slow deterioration of the kidneys during which the kidneys fail to rid the body of wastes. Diabetes is also the leading cause of limb amputation in the United States, and adults with diabetes are two to four times more likely to suffer from heart disease and stroke. The health care costs of treating the disease and its complications place an enormous burden on the diabetic and the nation as a whole. The average cost of treating diabetes can run from ten to twelve thousand dollars every year for the remainder of a diabetic's life, which is three to four times higher than the health care costs of a healthy person.

The primary characteristic of diabetes is the body's failure to metabolize glucose, the fuel the bloodstream carries to the cells of the body. After eating a meal, the body breaks down food into glucose, a sugar that circulates in the blood until needed by the body's cells. To metabolize glucose, the cell requires the hormone insulin, which is produced by the pancreas. For reasons scientists are just beginning to understand, insulin facilitates the process by which glucose can enter the "hungry" cell. In healthy people, the pancreas secretes insulin in response to a rise in blood sugar, and the insulin, in turn, helps the cells absorb the glucose the body needs for energy. With those who have diabetes, however, this process goes wrong. The body's cells are unable to absorb enough glucose, and the excess glucose remains in the bloodstream.

Although the primary symptom of all forms of diabetes is elevated blood glucose levels, the source of the problem varies with the type of diabetes a person develops. In type 1 diabetes, also known as juvenile diabetes because it most often appears in childhood, the beta cells that produce insulin have been destroyed by a disorder of the body's immune system. As a result, the pancreas is unable to supply the body with the insulin necessary to metabolize glucose. Given by injection, insulin reverses the wasting that accompanies type 1 diabetes. However, to manage the disease, victims of type 1 diabetes must inject the missing insulin for the remainder of their lives.

Type 2 diabetes, which accounts for 90 to 95 percent of all patients with diabetes, is a more complex disease. Although the body continues to produce insulin, the cells are unable to use it to absorb glucose. This phenomenon is known as insulin resistance, which precedes the onset of type 2 diabetes. When blood sugar levels skyrocket as more and more unmetabolized glucose enters the bloodstream, people with type 2 begin to develop symptoms because the cells of the body have difficulty obtaining the fuel they need to function.

In both forms of diabetes, the cells are deprived of their source of energy, and the muscle and nerve cells begin to slow, resulting in feelings of irritability and fatigue. Diabetics also often experience an insatiable thirst because the excess unmetabolized glucose that accumulates in the blood is sent to the kidneys, which require water to dilute the glucose. However, the most severe complications that accompany diabetes come when blood sugar levels remain elevated over time. These high glucose levels can exact a devastating toll on the body. The extra blood sugar slowly eats away at the body, damaging the tiny blood vessels in the eyes and nerves. Diabetes also forces the kidneys to work overtime, and without treatment, the kidneys ultimately lose their ability to function. In addition, for reasons scientists are just beginning to uncover, the excess glucose also damages the cardiovascular system, leading to heart disease and stroke.

Although researchers remain uncertain about exactly what causes the resistance to insulin that occurs in type 2 diabetes, studies have revealed factors that make some people more vulnerable to the disease than others. One of these factors is genetic. Diabetes runs in families, and minority populations seem to be especially susceptible. African Americans, Native Americans, and Hispanics, for example, are almost twice as likely to develop type 2 diabetes than whites. Environmental factors, however, also appear to play a significant role in vulnerability to type 2 diabetes. Research reveals that although as much as 85 percent of the population carries the diabetes gene, having the gene only increases the risk of developing type 2 diabetes by about 25 percent. However, when people genetically predisposed to the disease gain weight, their risk increases dramatically. Researchers continue to try to understand the exact nature of the relationship between obesity and diabetes, but the practical conclusion is that what makes people overweight—lack of exercise and a high-calorie diet—also puts them at risk for diabetes.

Sanford Garfield, a specialist with the National Institutes of Health, attributes the dramatic increase in the incidence of type 2 diabetes to what he calls "the McDonald's syndrome." More and more Americans eat unhealthy diets, gain weight, and have become more sedentary. As a result of this lifestyle, an increasing number of Americans have become obese, which increases their risk of developing type 2 diabetes. Evidence to support this theory comes from the fact that type 2 diabetes, once considered a disease that developed only in adulthood, has become more common among children who are obese. In the past, a majority of those who developed type 2 diabetes were more than thirty years of age. Now that more and more children are becoming obese, however, children as young as eight years old are developing the disease.

The key to managing both types of diabetes and avoiding the disease's complications is control of blood glucose levels. The Diabetes Control and Complications Trial (DCCT), a study conducted by the National Institute of Diabetes and Digestive and Kidney Diseases from 1983 to 1993, showed that keeping blood glucose levels as close to normal as possible slows the onset and progression of eye, kidney, and nerve diseases caused by diabetes. In fact, the DCCT demonstrated that any sustained lowering of blood glucose helps, even if the person has a history of poor control. With the development of home glucose monitoring systems, diabetics can measure their glucose levels throughout the day and adjust their diet or administer necessary insulin.

For type 2 diabetics, the best way to control blood glucose levels is to eat a low-fat, high-fiber, low-calorie diet and develop an exercise program. In addition, medications are available for type 2 diabetics that control blood sugar directly (biguanides), stimulate the production and release of insulin (sulfonylureas), or make the cells more sensitive to insulin (thiazolidinediones), but many type 2 diabetics can eliminate the need for drugs if they change their lifestyle. For reasons that are not yet clear, when people gain weight, the body becomes more resistant to insulin, and the pancreas works harder to circulate insulin. When type 2 diabetics lose weight, however, they can reverse the damage. Moreover, exercise makes the body's cells better able to absorb glucose, which keeps blood sugar levels in a healthier range. Research has also revealed that for those populations who are genetically predisposed to type 2 diabetes, a healthy diet and exercise can make a dramatic difference in whether they even develop the disease.

Although a healthy diet and exercise can improve the life of type 1 diabetics, because their pancreas has lost the ability to produce insulin, people who have type 1 diabetes must spend a lifetime pricking their fingers to test their blood sugar and injecting themselves with insulin, sometimes eight times daily. Unfortunately, insulin is not a cure for diabetes. People who develop type 1 diabetes require insulin therapy for survival, yet their blood glucose remains difficult to control, and most patients ultimately develop the devastating complications of this disease.

Because of the toll type 1 diabetes takes on those who develop the disease, the focus of research is to find a cure—a way to repair or replace the damaged insulin-producing beta cells of the pancreas. Once medical research improved organ transplant techniques in the 1960s, the first "cure" for type 1 diabetes was to replace the damaged pancreas with a healthy one. In 1966, the first pancreas transplant was used to treat type 1 diabetes. At that time, the rates of patient survival were low because the body's immune system attacked the new pancreas. However, in 1978, results were improved with the introduction of regimens of immunosuppressive drugs that inhibited the immune system's attack on the new organ. Patient outcomes were also improved when pancreatic transplants were accompanied by kidney transplants because of the complex relationship between the pancreas and the kidney and because the kidneys are often damaged in patients who have endured type 1 diabetes since childhood.

Although a pancreas transplant effectively cures diabetes in most cases, the procedure is not without risks. Transplants are extremely invasive and may be accompanied by the complications that can follow any surgery, including infection. The continued use of drugs to prevent the body's immune system from attacking the transplanted pancreas can complicate the body's ability to fight other infections, and these drugs have themselves been known to cause cancer, osteoporosis (bone disease), and the insulin resistance characteristic of type 2 diabetes. Moreover, despite their potential as a cure for type 1 diabetes, pancreatic transplants are reserved for only the most severe cases because few donor pancreases are available and the procedure is expensive.

Another less invasive option is transplantation of the islet cells that contain the insulin-producing beta cells. The human pancreas contains about 1 to 1.5 million islets, each containing about 2,500 cells, most of which are insulin-producing beta cells. When these cells are injected into the liver, they can function normally, secreting the insulin that maintains glucose levels. Major surgery is not required, and the procedure only takes from fifteen to forty-five minutes. Approximately 700,000 islet cells, each about the size of a grain of salt, are infused through a vein into the liver. The patient receives only a local anesthetic in the spot where a large needle is used to reach the portal vein that carries blood to the liver. The process is repeated within three months so that the liver will have nearly as many islet cells as a normal pancreas, about 1 million. Islet transplant is much cheaper than pancreas transplantation because it is an outpatient procedure, but because the procedure remains experimental, insurance companies do not yet cover the cost.

Between 1974 and 1996, more than 305 islet transplants were performed worldwide for type 1 diabetics. During that time 11 percent of the recipients remained independent of insulin injections for periods ranging from thirteen days to more than five years. However promising these results, researchers believed that they did not merit widespread use of islet transplantation. As with pancreas transplants, the immunosuppressive drugs that protect the islet cells from attack by the body's immune system increased the recipient's risk of infection and were sometimes even toxic to the very islets replaced.

A solution to the dangers posed by immunosuppressive drugs came in a study known as the Edmonton Protocol, led by James Shapiro at the University of Alberta in Edmonton. Shapiro used genetically engineered, steroid-free immunosuppressive drugs and achieved consistent insulin-independence in a small group of patients. Two years later, in 2002, the patients remained free of the life-threatening infections or cancer that had arisen with the use of other immunosuppressive drugs. Shapiro advises caution, however: "We have a gentler drug cocktail, but we really don't know what the long-term risks are going to be 20 to 30 years out." Moreover, some transplants have lost their effectiveness, and 30 percent of the initial patients have had to go back to using at least some insulin.

The enthusiasm generated by these results, however, provided hope of a miracle for the 1 million Americans who have type 1 diabetes. When the results of Shapiro's trials were published in the June 2000 issue of the *New England Journal of Medicine*, then President Bill Clinton announced a five-million-dollar program that established research centers at various locations throughout the United States to reproduce the Edmonton Protocol. The program has since become an international effort. If islet transplants prove successful for these patients over two to three years, the availability of the procedure may become more widespread.

The problem of the scarcity of islet tissue, however, remains. Only five hundred pancreases are available each year for islet cell transplants, and each patient requires cells from two pancreases. To resolve this problem, researchers are trying to develop other sources of tissue such as genetically engineered cells, stem cells, or pig pancreases. Those researchers at the forefront of these efforts agree that, notwithstanding the controversy and fear surrounding the use of these sources, despite their potential, human trials are years away.

Although new medical technologies are offering hope to both type 1 and type 2 diabetics, diabetes remains a lifelong disease with devastating and deadly complications. Unfortunately, despite medical advances, the number of those who develop diabetes, especially type 2, is increasing. The authors in *Diabetes: Contemporary Issues Companion*, explore the nature of diabetes, the impact of the epidemic, and directions in prevention and treatment, in articles that range from scientific surveys and editorials to personal accounts.

CHAPTER 1

THE NATURE OF DIABETES

THE NATURE OF DIABETES: AN OVERVIEW

National Institute of Diabetes and Digestive and Kidney Diseases

Diabetes is a leading cause of death and disability in the United States, and the percentage of the American population expected to develop diabetes is expected to rise to 8.9 percent by 2025, according to the National Institute of Diabetes and Digestive and Kidney Diseases (NIDDK). In the following selection, the NIDDK provides an overview of the nature and symptoms of the three main types of diabetes, the ways each is diagnosed and managed, and the impact and scope of the disease. The institute explains, for example, that diabetes affects the body's ability to pass energy-providing glucose into the bloodstream. According to the NIDDK, the body with type 1 diabetes stops producing the insulin that facilitates this process, while the body with type 2 diabetes produces insulin but cannot use it properly. Because of these differences, the institute reports, each form of diabetes presents different symptoms and requires different treatment. All forms of diabetes have serious, long-term complications at a tremendous cost to society, so the NIDDK and other organizations continue to conduct research to find better ways to treat diabetes and search for ways to prevent or even cure this debilitating disease. The NIDDK is a branch of the National Institutes of Health that conducts and supports research on diabetes and other serious diseases.

Almost everyone knows someone who has diabetes. More than 16 million people in the United States have diabetes mellitus—a serious, lifelong condition. Each year, about 800,000 people are diagnosed with diabetes.

What Is Diabetes?

Diabetes is a disorder of metabolism—the way our bodies use digested food for growth and energy. Most of the food we eat is broken down

From National Institute of Diabetes and Digestive and Kidney Diseases, *Diabetes Overview*, National Diabetes Information Clearinghouse, November 1998, updated July 2001.

into glucose, the form of sugar in the blood. Glucose is the main source of fuel for the body.

After digestion, glucose passes into the bloodstream, where it is used by cells for growth and energy. For glucose to get into cells, insulin must be present. Insulin is a hormone produced by the pancreas, a large gland behind the stomach.

When we eat, the pancreas is supposed to automatically produce the right amount of insulin to move glucose from blood into our cells. In people with diabetes, however, the pancreas either produces little or no insulin, or the cells do not respond appropriately to the insulin that is produced. Glucose builds up in the blood, overflows into the urine, and passes out of the body. Thus, the body loses its main source of fuel even though the blood contains large amounts of glucose.

What Are the Types of Diabetes?

The three main types of diabetes are
- Type 1 diabetes
- Type 2 diabetes
- Gestational diabetes

Type 1 diabetes is an autoimmune disease. An autoimmune disease results when the body's system for fighting infection (the immune system) turns against a part of the body. In diabetes, the immune system attacks the insulin-producing beta cells in the pancreas and destroys them. The pancreas then produces little or no insulin. Someone with type 1 diabetes needs to take insulin daily to live.

As of this writing, scientists do not know exactly what causes the body's immune system to attack the beta cells, but they believe that both genetic factors and environmental factors, possibly viruses, are involved. Type 1 diabetes accounts for about 5 to 10 percent of diagnosed diabetes in the United States.

Type 1 diabetes develops most often in children and young adults, but the disorder can appear at any age. Symptoms of type 1 diabetes usually develop over a short period, although beta cell destruction can begin years earlier.

Symptoms include increased thirst and urination, constant hunger, weight loss, blurred vision, and extreme fatigue. If not diagnosed and treated with insulin, a person can lapse into a life-threatening diabetic coma, also known as diabetic ketoacidosis.

Type 2 Diabetes

The most common form of diabetes is type 2 diabetes. About 90 to 95 percent of people with diabetes have type 2, and one-third of them have not been diagnosed. This form of diabetes usually develops in adults age 40 and older and is most common in adults over age 55. About 80 percent of people with type 2 diabetes are overweight. Type 2 diabetes is often part of a metabolic syndrome that includes obesity, elevated blood pressure, and high levels of blood lipids. Unfortunately, as more children become overweight, type 2 diabetes is becoming more common in young people.

When type 2 diabetes is diagnosed, the pancreas is usually producing enough insulin, but, for unknown reasons, the body cannot use the insulin effectively, a condition called insulin resistance. After several years, insulin production decreases. The result is the same as for type 1 diabetes—glucose builds up in the blood and the body cannot make efficient use of its main source of fuel.

The symptoms of type 2 diabetes develop gradually. They are not as sudden in onset as in type 1 diabetes. Some people have no symptoms. Symptoms may include fatigue or nausea, frequent urination, unusual thirst, weight loss, blurred vision, frequent infections, and slow healing of wounds or sores.

Gestational Diabetes

Gestational diabetes develops only during pregnancy. Like type 2 diabetes, it occurs more often in African Americans, American Indians, Hispanic Americans, and people with a family history of diabetes. Though it usually disappears after delivery, the mother is at increased risk of getting type 2 diabetes later in life.

Diagnosing Diabetes

The fasting plasma glucose test is the preferred test for diagnosing type 1 or type 2 diabetes. However, a diagnosis of diabetes is made for any one of three positive tests, with a second positive test on a different day:

- A random plasma glucose value (taken any time of day) of 200 milligrams per deciliter (mg/dL) or more, along with the presence of diabetes symptoms.
- A plasma glucose value of 126 mg/dL or more, after a person has fasted for 8 hours.
- An oral glucose tolerance test (OGTT) plasma glucose value of 200 mg/dL or more in the blood sample, taken 2 hours after a person has consumed a drink containing 75 grams of glucose dissolved in water. This test, taken in a laboratory or the doctor's office, measures plasma glucose at timed intervals over a 3-hour period.

Gestational diabetes is diagnosed based on plasma glucose values measured during the OGTT. Glucose levels are normally lower during pregnancy, so the threshold values for diagnosis of diabetes in pregnancy are lower. If a woman has two plasma glucose values meeting or exceeding any of the following numbers, she has gestational diabetes: a fasting plasma glucose level of 95 mg/dL, a 1-hour level of 180 mg/dL, a 2-hour level of 155 mg/dL, or a 3-hour level of 140 mg/dL.

People with impaired glucose metabolism, a state between "normal" and "diabetes," are at risk for developing diabetes, heart attacks, and strokes. There are two forms of impaired glucose metabolism.

A person has impaired fasting glucose (IFG) when fasting plasma glucose is 110 to 125 mg/dL. This level is higher than normal but less than the level indicating a diagnosis of diabetes. Approximately 13.4 million people in the United States, or about 7 percent of the population, have IFG.

Impaired glucose tolerance (IGT) means that blood glucose during the oral glucose tolerance test is higher than normal but not high enough for a diagnosis of diabetes. IGT is diagnosed when the glucose level is 141 to 199 mg/dL 2 hours after a person is given a drink containing 75 grams of glucose.

The Scope and Impact of Diabetes

Diabetes is widely recognized as one of the leading causes of death and disability in the United States. According to death certificate data, diabetes contributed to the deaths of more than 193,140 people in 1996.

Diabetes is associated with long-term complications that affect almost every part of the body. The disease often leads to blindness, heart and blood vessel disease, strokes, kidney failure, amputations, and nerve damage. Uncontrolled diabetes can complicate pregnancy, and birth defects are more common in babies born to women with diabetes.

In 1997, diabetes cost the United States $98 billion. Indirect costs, including disability payments, time lost from work, and premature death, totaled $54 billion; direct medical costs for diabetes care, including hospitalizations, medical care, and treatment supplies, totaled $44 billion.

Who Gets Diabetes?

Diabetes is not contagious. People cannot "catch" it from each other. However, certain factors can increase the risk of developing diabetes.

Type 1 diabetes occurs equally among males and females, but is more common in whites than in nonwhites. Data from the World Health Organization's Multinational Project for Childhood Diabetes indicate that type 1 diabetes is rare in most African, American Indian, and Asian populations. However, some northern European countries, including Finland and Sweden, have high rates of type 1 diabetes. The reasons for these differences are not known.

Type 2 diabetes is more common in older people, especially in people who are overweight, and occurs more often in African Americans, American Indians, Asian and Pacific Islander Americans, and Hispanic Americans. On average, non-Hispanic African Americans are 1.7 times more likely to have diabetes than non-Hispanic whites of the same age. Hispanic Americans are nearly twice as likely to have diabetes as non-Hispanic whites. American Indians have the highest rates of diabetes in the world. Among the Pima Indians living in Arizona, for example, half of all adults have type 2 diabetes.

The prevalence of diabetes in the United States is likely to increase for several reasons. First, a large segment of the population is aging. Also, Hispanic Americans and other minority groups make up the fastest-growing segment of the U.S. population. Finally, Americans are increasingly overweight and sedentary. According to recent estimates, the prevalence of diabetes in the United States is predicted to be 8.9 percent of the population by 2025.

Managing Diabetes

Before the discovery of insulin in 1921, everyone with type 1 diabetes died within a few years after diagnosis. Although insulin is not considered a cure, its discovery was the first major breakthrough in diabetes treatment.

Today, healthy eating, physical activity, and insulin via injection or an insulin pump are the basic therapies for type 1 diabetes. The amount of insulin must be balanced with food intake and daily activities. Blood glucose levels must be closely monitored through frequent blood glucose checking.

Healthy eating, physical activity, and blood glucose testing are the basic management tools for type 2 diabetes. In addition, many people with type 2 diabetes require oral medication and insulin to control their blood glucose levels.

People with diabetes must take responsibility for their day-to-day care. Much of the daily care involves keeping blood glucose levels from going too low or too high. When blood glucose levels drop too low from certain diabetes medicines—a condition known as hypoglycemia—a person can become nervous, shaky, and confused. Judgment can be impaired. If blood glucose falls too low, a person can faint.

A person can also become ill if blood glucose levels rise too high, a condition known as hyperglycemia.

People with diabetes should see a doctor who helps them learn to manage their diabetes and monitors their diabetes control. An endocrinologist is one type of doctor who may specialize in diabetes care. In addition, people with diabetes often see ophthalmologists for eye examinations, podiatrists for routine foot care, and dietitians and diabetes educators to help teach the skills of day-to-day diabetes management.

Controlling Glucose Levels

The goal of diabetes management is to keep blood glucose levels as close to the normal range as safely possible. A recent major study, the Diabetes Control and Complications Trial (DCCT), sponsored by the National Institute of Diabetes and Digestive and Kidney Diseases (NIDDK), showed that keeping blood glucose levels as close to normal as safely possible reduces the risk of developing major complications of type 1 diabetes.

The 10-year study, completed in 1993, included 1,441 people with type 1 diabetes. The study compared the effect of two treatment approaches—intensive management and standard management—on the development and progression of eye, kidney, and nerve complications of diabetes. Intensive treatment aimed at keeping hemoglobin A-1-c as close to normal (6 percent) as possible. Hemoglobin A-1-c reflects average blood sugar over a 2- to 3-month period. Researchers found that study participants who maintained lower levels of blood glucose through intensive management had significantly lower rates of these complications. More recently, a followup study of DCCT participants showed that the ability of intensive control to lower the complications of diabetes persists up to 4 years after the trial ended.

The United Kingdom Prospective Diabetes Study, a European study completed in 1998, showed that intensive control of blood glucose and blood pressure reduced the risk of blindness, kidney disease, stroke, and heart attack in people with type 2 diabetes.

The Status of Diabetes Research

NIDDK conducts research in its own laboratories and supports a great deal of basic and clinical research in medical centers and hospitals throughout the United States. It also gathers and analyzes statistics about diabetes. Other Institutes at the National Institutes of Health (NIH) conduct and support research on diabetes-related eye diseases, heart and vascular complications, pregnancy, and dental problems.

Other Government agencies that sponsor diabetes programs are the Centers for Disease Control and Prevention, the Indian Health Service, the Health Resources and Services Administration, the Department of Veterans Affairs, and the Department of Defense.

Many organizations outside of the Government support diabetes research and education activities. These organizations include the American Diabetes Association, the Juvenile Diabetes Foundation International, and the American Association of Diabetes Educators.

Advances in diabetes research have led to better ways to manage diabetes and treat its complications. Major advances include

- The development of a quick-acting insulin analog.
- Better ways to monitor blood glucose and for people with diabetes to check their own blood glucose levels.
- Development of external insulin pumps that deliver insulin, replacing daily injections.
- Laser treatment for diabetic eye disease, reducing the risk of blindness.
- Successful transplantation of kidneys and pancreas in people whose own kidneys fail because of diabetes.
- Better ways of managing diabetes in pregnant women, improving chances of successful outcomes.
- New drugs to treat type 2 diabetes and better ways to manage

this form of diabetes through weight control.

- Evidence that intensive management of blood glucose reduces and may prevent development of diabetes complications.
- Demonstration that antihypertensive drugs called ACE (angiotensin-converting enzyme) inhibitors prevent or delay kidney failure in people with diabetes.
- Promising results with islet transplantation for type 1 diabetes reported by the University of Alberta in Canada. A nationwide clinical trial funded by the NIH and the Juvenile Diabetes Foundation is currently trying to replicate the Canadian advance.

What Will the Future Bring?

In the future, it may be possible to administer insulin through inhalers, a pill, or a patch. Devices are also being developed that can monitor blood glucose levels without having to prick a finger to get a blood sample.

Researchers continue to search for the cause or causes of diabetes and ways to prevent and cure the disorder. Scientists are looking for genes that may be involved in type 1 or type 2 diabetes. Some genetic markers for type 1 diabetes have been identified, and it is now possible to screen relatives of people with type 1 diabetes to see if they are at risk.

The Diabetes Prevention Trial—Type 1, sponsored by NIDDK, identifies relatives at risk for developing type 1 diabetes and treats them with low doses of insulin or with oral insulin-like agents in the hope of preventing type 1 diabetes. Similar research is under way at other medical centers throughout the world. . . .

Transplantation of the pancreas or insulin-producing beta cells offers the best hope of cure for people with type 1 diabetes. Some pancreas transplants have been successful. However, people who have transplants must take powerful drugs to prevent rejection of the transplanted organ. These drugs are costly and may eventually cause other health problems.

Scientists are working to develop less harmful drugs and better methods of transplanting beta cells to prevent rejection by the body. Using techniques of bioengineering, researchers are also trying to create artificial beta cells that secrete insulin in response to increased glucose levels in the blood.

Researchers at the University of Alberta in Edmonton, Canada, announced promising results with islet transplantation in seven patients with type 1 diabetes. At the time of the report in the *New England Journal of Medicine*, all seven patients who had received the transplant remained free of insulin injections up to 14 months after the procedure.

A clinical trial funded by the NIH and the Juvenile Diabetes Foundation will try to replicate the Edmonton advance. With the insights gained from this trial and other studies, scientists hope to further refine methods of islet harvesting and transplantation and learn more about the immune processes that affect rejection and acceptance of transplanted islets.

For type 2 diabetes, the focus is on ways to prevent diabetes. Preventive approaches include identifying people at high risk for the disorder and encouraging them to lose weight, be more physically active, and follow a healthy eating plan. The Diabetes Prevention Program, another NIDDK project, focuses on preventing the disorder in high-risk populations, such as people with impaired fasting glucose, African Americans, Alaska Natives, American Indians, Asian and Pacific Islander Americans, Hispanic Americans, or women who have had gestational diabetes.

Several new drugs have been developed to treat type 2 diabetes. By using the oral diabetes medications now available, many people can control blood glucose levels without insulin injections. Studies are under way to determine how best to use these drugs to manage type 2 diabetes. Scientists also are investigating strategies for weight loss in people with type 2 diabetes.

DIABETES: A GLOBAL EPIDEMIC

Paul Zimmet

According to the World Health Organization, the number of people with diabetes will double from 150 million to an estimated 300 million by 2025, writes Paul Zimmet in the following selection. Diabetes has become a global epidemic with severe economic consequences, Zimmet claims, particularly for developing countries. Zimmet explains, for example, that many people from developing countries have a genetic susceptibility to diabetes. Moreover, he asserts, the modernization that accompanies globalization has caused them to adopt the sedentary lifestyle and unhealthy diet of modern nations. Because type 2 diabetes is linked to obesity, lack of exercise, and poor diet, populations of developing nations will bear the burden of the diabetes epidemic, argues Zimmet. Diabetes, he observes, is a global lifestyle problem that could be prevented with education about the importance of a proper diet and exercise. Zimmet is the director of the International Diabetes Institute, head of the World Health Organization Collaborating Centre for the Epidemiology of Diabetes Mellitus and Health Promotion for Noncommunicable Disease Control, and professor of diabetes at Monash University in Melbourne, Australia.

"The world will witness human calamity of unthinkable proportions destined to strain social and economic resources"

This statement by Professor Anuar Zaini, one of Asia's foremost diabetologists, encapsulates well the threat we face from the spectacular rise in the global prevalence of diabetes mellitus. The number of cases has reached epidemic proportions, and continues to increase sharply. The World Health Organization (WHO) predicts that the number of people with diabetes will double within just one generation, from 150 million in 2001 to an estimated 300 million in 2025.

And yet we are ill-prepared to tackle this epidemic effectively. As the International Diabetes Federation (IDF) states in its Diabetes Atlas 2000 report: "Many governments and public health planners remain

From "The Rise and Rise of Diabetes," by Paul Zimmet, *Pathways: The Novartis Journal,* July 2001. Copyright © 2001 by Excerpta Medica. Reprinted with permission.

largely unaware of the current magnitude or, more importantly, the future potential for increases in diabetes and its serious complications in their own countries." Clearly, this situation must be rectified, not least because the economic burden of the diabetes epidemic—the direct costs of healthcare plus the indirect costs from loss of productivity and from premature morbidity and mortality—could cripple the budgets of some nations, particularly developing countries.

The Prevalence of Key Risk Factors

Most of the increase as of July 2001, and the projected increase, involves type 2 diabetes, formerly known as non-insulin-dependent diabetes mellitus (NIDDM). This is the most common form of the disease, accounting for up to 95 percent of all cases and occurring mainly in adults. But why is the prevalence of type 2 diabetes rising so alarmingly? The answer lies in the increasing prevalence of its key risk factors, which include obesity, a sedentary lifestyle and an unhealthy diet.

The link between obesity and type 2 diabetes is especially strong, so strong that some specialists have suggested using the term "diabesity" to better describe the current epidemic. Indeed, there are believed to be more than 250 million obese adults worldwide. The risk of developing type 2 diabetes rises with increasing body weight, and is about 5–10 times greater in people classified as obese (having a body mass index of 30 or above) than in those with a 'normal' weight (body mass index under 25). Early in 2001 researchers in the US identified a hormone called resistin, which might possibly explain the obesity-diabetes link at a biochemical level. They found that in mice (the hormone is present in humans but has not yet been studied to any extent) obesity induced elevated blood levels of resistin, which in turn induced insulin resistance and glucose intolerance.

At a global level the diabesity epidemic is being fueled by rapid cultural and social changes. It is occurring concurrently with increased urbanization, and with a modernization (or "Westernization") of lifestyle. In many countries, traditional lifestyles and dietary patterns are disappearing as people adapt to living in the more industrialized, urban environments that are brought about by the socioeconomic forces of globalization. People all over the world are living longer, and are more likely to have a relatively sedentary lifestyle, a high-calorie diet, and to be overweight or obese.

The extent to which this results in type 2 diabetes within populations is determined by the level of genetic susceptibility. Although diabetes affects people of all races and classes, we know that certain ethnic groups have a greater susceptibility to developing type 2 diabetes than others. This increased susceptibility was first noted among people in the Pacific and Indian Ocean regions, and more recently in the rest of Asia and the Middle East. It also applies to disadvantaged communities in developed nations, including native Americans, African Americans and Hispanic populations in the US; native Canadians; Aborigines and Torres Strait Islanders in Australia; and Polynesians in New Zealand. Their greater genetic susceptibility to type 2 diabetes is being unmasked by the changing environmental and behavioral factors such as a poor or unbalanced diet and a sedentary lifestyle.

This suggests that the developing world will bear most of the burden of the diabesity epidemic in the future, and this is confirmed by the WHO figures. While the prevalence of adult diabetes in developed countries is expected to rise by a total of 41 percent between 1995 and 2025 (a very large increase in its own right), the prevalence of the disease in developing countries is predicted to rise by 170 percent over the same period.

The Mauritius Microcosm

One of the best indications of the scale of the problem facing much of the developing world has come from extensive research on the Indian Ocean island of Mauritius. The island has a population of 1.3 million, and includes people of Asian Indian, Chinese and black (Creole) descent. As these groups constitute nearly two-thirds of the world's population, what happens on Mauritius is in many ways a microcosm of the global situation. Surveys on the island in 1987 revealed a high diabetes prevalence, of about 10–13 percent in each ethnic group (rising to 20–30 percent in those aged 45–74 years). A follow-up study in 1998 showed that the number of people with diabetes had risen by 33 percent in the intervening 11 years. Almost 20 percent of the population over 30 years of age now have the condition. These results, extrapolated to parts of India, China and Africa where modernization and industrialization are occurring, account for much of the huge increase in the number of cases of type 2 diabetes that is being predicted.

The Mauritius research has uncovered the highest yet reported prevalence of type 2 diabetes among people of Chinese extraction. This, combined with a doubling in prevalence among Singaporean Chinese between 1984 and 1998, and high rates in Hong Kong and Taiwan, provides an alarming indication of the magnitude of the future epidemic in China itself. Until relatively recently the overall prevalence of type 2 diabetes in China was less than 1 percent. Studies have since revealed a three-fold increase in prevalence in certain areas over the past two decades. Significantly, if the rate of diabetes in China were to become just half of the current rate in Taiwan, the number of people with the disease would increase from about 10 million in 2000 to over 32 million by 2010.

Type 2 Developing at a Younger Age

The falling age of onset of type 2 diabetes is an important factor influencing the future burden of the disease. Type 2 diabetes was once considered to be a disease that developed only in adults, usually after the age of 40 years, and indeed it used to be known as adult-onset diabetes (with type 1, the form of the disease traditionally seen mainly in children, known as juvenile-onset diabetes). In many populations, however, especially those at high risk of type 2 diabetes such as native Americans and indigenous Australians, we are increasingly seeing disease onset in people aged below 30. The increase in type 2 diabetes among children, adolescents and younger adults is due mainly to lifestyle factors and rising rates of obesity in these groups. Among children in Japan, type 2 diabetes is already far more common than type 1 diabetes, accounting for 80 percent of cases of diabetes in childhood. This situation may perhaps be related to observations that Japanese Americans do not need to gain nearly as much weight as other ethnic groups to develop diabetes.

More and more people worldwide are therefore developing type 2 diabetes, and they are developing it at younger ages. What are the implications of this for society? First, the burden on primary, secondary and tertiary healthcare services is becoming greater, as rising numbers of affected individuals require the long-term treatment and support necessary to lead a normal life. The direct medical costs of diabetes are significant—a study in eight European countries showed that type 2 diabetes accounted for 3–6 percent of overall healthcare expenditure, while in the US the figure is as high as 12 percent. Most of the medical costs of the disease relate to the management and treatment of diabetic complications, with hospitalization the single largest category of costs.

The indirect costs of the disease accrued through loss of productivity to society can be even larger than the direct costs, and will only increase further with the downward shift in the age of onset, as a greater proportion of the workforce becomes disabled by the condition. Recent figures from the US show that the total economic costs of diabetes rose from $20.4 billion in 1987 to $98 billion in 1997 ($44 billion direct costs and $54 billion indirect costs). Also in the US, the number of workers permanently disabled because of diabetes increased by more than 50 percent between 1992 and 1997, from 47,800 to 74,927. Accurate cost estimates for developing countries are not yet available, but there is no doubt that the diabesity epidemic is likely to have devastating economic consequences in the near future.

Coping with the Epidemic

Clinically, early detection of diabetes provides an opportunity to reduce the progression of microvascular or macrovascular disease caused by asymptomatic hyperglycemia [abnormally high blood glucose]. Yet currently, about 20 percent of people already have complications by the time they are diagnosed with type 2 diabetes. More widespread screening for diabetes, to detect cases as early as possible, should be encouraged.

Several recent landmark studies, including the United Kingdom Prospective Diabetes Study (UKPDS) and Micro-Hope studies, have shown that the risk of complications can be substantially reduced, and progression of existing problems slowed, through improved metabolic control and reduction of key risk factors such as dyslipidemia [abnormal cholesterol levels] and hypertension. This "complete approach" to the management of diabetes has the potential to greatly improve the prognosis for patients with diabetes.

The most promising way to curb the impact of the diabetes epidemic, however, must be through primary prevention. The most potent currently recognized environmental risk factors for type 2 diabetes—diet, physical activity and obesity—are all modifiable through lifestyle intervention. Encouraging people from an early age to eat healthily and exercise regularly could have beneficial effects in the long-term on the prevalence of diabetes.

But it will take a much more integrated approach to have a significant impact on the epidemic. We need to begin viewing type 2 diabetes not only as a disease, but also as a symptom of a much larger global problem—the effect on human health of environmental and lifestyle changes. Type 2 diabetes is not the only "Western" disease on the increase globally—cancer, coronary heart disease and cerebrovascular disease are also becoming increasingly prevalent for similar reasons—but it is one of the most obvious manifestations of the major social and public health problem facing the world. The task of preventing and controlling these noncommunicable, lifestyle-related diseases does not lie solely with the medical community. The WHO's 1999 World Health Report made it clear that the responsibility for global health also lies with public and social planners, private enterprise, economists and politicians.

It is not too late for nations to develop highly integrated policies for education and intervention. For example, policies for consumer education that promote a healthy diet could be reinforced by legislative changes such as increased taxation of certain 'unhealthy' foods. This is obviously a very complex area, fraught with potential hazards. Because of this, a priority should be the establishment of a multidisciplinary international task force representing all parties that can help reverse the underlying socioeconomic causes of the problem. The international diabetes and public health communities must begin lobbying and mobilizing politicians and international nongovernmental agencies to address the issues that have led to the type 2 diabetes and non-communicable disease epidemic.

We can resolve this problem, but it will require a unique coordinated approach unlike anything tried before. This is the real challenge for us all today.

Genetics, Gender, and the Diabetic Family

Rowan Hillson

In the following excerpt from her book *Practical Diabetes Care*, Dr. Rowan Hillson discusses the impact diabetes may have on families and suggests strategies the family can employ to cope with the disease. The author explains, for example, that diabetes can create fear and anxiety among family members, so the entire family must learn about the nature and treatment of diabetes. The author also reveals the varied impact diabetes may have on women and men. According to Hillson, diabetic women who choose to have children may risk complications during pregnancy and must consider the possibility that their own health may deteriorate while they are raising their children. Both diabetic mothers and fathers, she writes, often neglect their own health in an effort to provide for their children. However, with the support of medical personnel, the author writes, the diabetic family can learn to cope with the complications of the disease. Hillson is a consultant physician of diabetic care at the Hillingdon Hospital in Uxbridge, Middlesex, England.

Diabetes in one family member influences all the others, indeed, some family members may subsequently develop diabetes themselves. It is important that family and friends realize that diabetes is not infectious. The risk of inheriting diabetes differs between insulin-dependent diabetes mellitus (IDDM) and non-insulin-dependent diabetes mellitus (NIDDM), and is difficult to quantify as the development of diabetes appears to be an amalgam of genetics and environment. Published estimations vary.

The Inheritance of Diabetes

An identical twin has a 30–50 per cent chance of developing IDDM if his twin has it. The sibling of someone with IDDM has about an 8 per cent chance of developing diabetes. A child has a 1–2 per cent chance of developing diabetes if his mother has it and a 6 per cent chance if his father has it. If both parents have IDDM, the risk is 30 per cent. These figures should be compared with the frequency of IDDM in the population as a whole which is 0.25 per cent.

The chance of inheriting NIDDM is harder to assess as some individuals do not develop the disease until their 80s. There is virtually 100 per cent concordance [presence of a trait] of diabetes in identical twins. About 25 per cent of the relatives of someone with NIDDM have had, have, or eventually develop diabetes. If one parent has NIDDM about 15 per cent of their children will eventually develop it; if both parents have NIDDM the risk may be as high as 75 per cent. The frequency in the population as a whole is 1–2 per cent.

The Impact of Diabetes on the Family

The discovery of diabetes in a child can cause major stresses within a family. If a parent has it, there may be much self-blame. The pattern of family life may be interrupted by the mechanics of diabetes care. Other siblings may feel left out as much attention and anxiety is lavished upon their brother or sister. They may also be frightened, especially if their sibling was rushed to hospital very ill. 'Is Johnny going to die? Am I going to catch diabetes?'

If an adult develops diabetes the impact upon the family is variable. Some self-sufficient couples cope well:

Alexander developed diabetes days before his wife was due to deliver their first child. Within three days the couple had bought a selection of diabetes books, learned how to master his treatment and blood testing, and had the satisfaction of seeing his blood glucose begin to fall. By the time the child was born Alexander's blood glucose was normal and both parents became fully occupied in caring for their baby daughter.

Others react differently:

Ernest was horrified when his wife developed diabetes. The elderly couple had experienced no serious illnesses before. He took over her diet, her treatment, and even talked for her during consultations. Doris appeared to know nothing about her diabetes and the diabetes team were never able to persuade her to take any interest in her condition. When Doris developed an infection her husband tried to manage her diabetes alone at home for some days and she was seriously ill and grossly hyperglycaemic when she was finally admitted. Ernest spent every day in hospital with her. He became exhausted and finally confessed that he was having chest pain. He was admitted and it was some weeks before both were fit enough for discharge.

In some families the diabetes diet is seen as very unusual. The person with diabetes may have to sit watching everyone else eat bacon, sausage, and chips followed by chocolate whip and sugary biscuits while she eats chicken salad and fruit. Women are more likely to change their diet to a diabetes one if their husband has diabetes than vice versa. As the diabetes diet is that recommended for the population at large the whole family should adopt it.

Diabetes may become an open, accepted part of family life, a weapon or defence, or an enemy which causes disability or financial disaster. The person with diabetes needs the full support of his or her family. If the patient agrees, close family members should be encouraged to meet the diabetes team and learn more about diabetes. The general practitioner (GP) and practice team can provide diabetes education, and support family members as well as the patient.

For optimal care, it is essential that people with diabetes live in accommodation in which they can readily maintain a high standard of personal hygiene, where they can keep their medication and equipment secure and where they are not exposed to extremes of temperature, or infection due, for example, to poor food storage or infestation. Every person with diabetes must have a telephone or be able to summon help if taken ill at home, 24 hours a day. . . .

The Impact on Women

All the changes of womanhood can influence, and be influenced by, diabetes.

The hormonal changes preceding and during menstruation can cause both hypoglycaemia [abnormal decrease of sugar in the blood] and hyperglycaemia [excess of sugar in the blood] in different individuals. The most frequent change is hyperglycaemia, on the last day or so premenstrually or, most often, during the first two days of bleeding. Some women are hypoglycaemic premenstrually or as the bleeding subsides. In others unpredictable oscillations in glycaemic balance appear to be the problem. Some women increase their insulin for the first two days of bleeding. Hyperglycaemia can cause menstrual irregularity or amenorrhoea [abnormal absence of menstruation], especially in untreated diabetes.

Vaginal thrush is a common presenting feature in diabetic women and is often difficult to eradicate. The perineal soreness and irritation can be extremely distressing and may cause irritability and sleep disturbance. Good glycaemic control improves the chances of cure using standard antifungals. The partner should be treated as well. Herpes simplex and herpes zoster, and vaginal warts all appear more common in women with diabetes. Urinary tract infections can add to the woman's misery and it may co-exist with candidiasis [fungus infection]. . . .

The Diabetic Pregnancy

Diabetic women have near-normal fertility unless they have persistently high blood glucose levels, or have renal impairment. Even then, conception can occur. Teenage girls should know that it is important to plan pregnancy when they do decide to have a family and that contraception should be used, if necessary, until then.

Congenital malformations used to be two to three times as common in diabetic pregnancies as in the general population. Then it was found that malformations were most likely in women with hyperglycaemia in the first 8 weeks of pregnancy (for example women whose haemoglobin A1 was ever 10 per cent). Maintenance of strict normoglycaemia reduces the likelihood of congenital malformation to near that of the non-diabetic population. . . .

The woman's fitness to withstand pregnancy and her prospects of healthy survival during the years in which her child needs her most must also be considered. Women with severe tissue damage are surviving pregnancy with normal infants, but this requires nine months of very intensive effort, and the harsh reality is that they may become severely disabled or die before their child grows up. Retinopathy can worsen dramatically in pregnancy and fundoscopy [examination of the eyes] should be part of the pre-pregnancy screen as should assessment of renal function. Renal failure may also worsen considerably during pregnancy and such women should be managed jointly by obstetrician, renal physician, and diabetologist from pre-pregnancy onwards. . . .

In a diabetic pregnancy, the risks to the patient and fetus include pregnancy-induced hypertension, polyhydramnios [too much fluid around the fetus], ketoacidosis [a series of complications that result when the body cannot use glucose as fuel], fetal malformation, poor fetal growth, macrosomia [having an unusually large body], sudden intrauterine death, respiratory distress syndrome, and post-partum hypoglycaemia (for both). These complications can be reduced by intensive diabetes and obstetric management but some women who have been normoglycaemic throughout pregnancy still have macrosomic babies.

One of the difficulties with care of the pregnant diabetic woman is that there is no consensus about the precise blood glucose levels to aim for, the process of obstetric care or the type or timing of delivery. The most important factor appears to be frequent care by a team experienced in the management of diabetes in pregnancy, with close attention to detail, and 24-hour availability of immediate help (by telephone or in person) if problems arise.

Diabetes may arise during pregnancy and is especially likely in the third trimester. . . . Once diagnosed, women with gestational diabetes are treated like any other pregnant diabetic woman. After delivery, glucose tolerance may revert to normal, or remain impaired. Up to 60 per cent of women with gestational diabetes may eventually develop permanent diabetes. This is especially likely in Asian women. The maintenance of a diabetic diet and regular exercise may delay or prevent the reappearance of diabetes. There is a high likelihood of gestational diabetes in further pregnancies. . . .

Motherhood and Menopause

Women sometimes forget about themselves as they rush around, cooking, cleaning, picking Johnny up from nursery school, delivering Suzanne to ballet, and more. It is even harder work if the woman has an additional paid job. The diabetes can be the last item on the agenda and the aim may be seen as 'keeping a little sugary to avoid hypoglycaemia and not testing too much because I'm busy.' The diet may be erratic, including remnants from the children's plates. Of course, they know what they ought to be doing but this is just until the children are older. A family of two can occupy a woman for 18–20 years—long enough to develop all the complications of diabetes. Mothers should be encouraged to give themselves some time for daily body maintenance—perhaps at a time when their partner is at home and can look after the children. . . .

Blood glucose balance occasionally becomes erratic during the menopause although afterwards the insulin requirement may fall. This may not apply if the woman is given hormone replacement therapy. There are several views on this, but providing the treatment is given in truly 'replacement' doses, i.e., physiological rather than pharmacological, it seems sensible to apply the same criteria for initiating hormone replacement therapy as in nondiabetic women.

The Impact on Men

The diabetic father is under many of the same pressures as the diabetic mother: he may be the one looking after the children. In many cases, he may be the breadwinner. They may worry that their diabetes is going to stop them working and make them let their family down. As with working women, they may be working so hard, that they neglect themselves and their diabetes. They may ignore check-ups because they do not wish to take time off work. It may be difficult to contact them but they may be prepared to attend an evening or Saturday clinic. Being self-employed can be particularly stressful.

Untreated diabetes or hyperglycaemia can reduce libido temporarily. Diabetic men may also develop candidal infection: balanitis. Both the man and his partner should be treated with antifungals. As in women, the critical factor is returning the blood glucose toward normal. Fertility is not impaired and there appears to be no problem for the fetus if the father has hyperglycaemia at conception.

Approximately one in three men with diabetes may experience impotence, either temporarily or permanently. Impotence may be under-reported as the ambience of many diabetic clinics or busy surgeries is not always conducive to such sensitive discussions. Bearing in mind that it may have taken considerable courage on the patient's part to reveal this symptom, any mention of impotence should be followed up, if necessary at another appointment with appropriate privacy and time, and preferably with his partner.

The first step is to define the patient's problem. Impotence is the inability to develop and maintain a penile erection sufficient for sexual intercourse. Although some men with diabetes do have permanent impotence associated with diabetic tissue damage, many have reversible impotence. Reversible factors, or those suggesting another condition requiring investigation and treatment should be sought, but a final decision that the impotence is due to diabetes does not mean that the patient and his partner cannot be helped.

THE LINK BETWEEN ETHNICITY, TYPE 2 DIABETES, AND HEART DISEASE

Heart Disease Weekly

Heart disease, the most deadly complication of diabetes, is the leading cause of death for African Americans and Hispanics, write the editors of *Heart Disease Weekly*. Unfortunately, the authors observe, many among these at-risk populations are unaware of the connection between diabetes and heart disease, and tests that measure the blood sugar levels of these diabetic patients reveal that a substantial number do not effectively manage their disease. In order to control the epidemic of diabetic heart disease, the authors explain, education of these ethnic groups is critical. *Heart Disease Weekly* is a business and consumer newsletter that covers issues relating to the human heart and coronary disease.

According to a survey released by the Association of Black Cardiologists (ABC), more than 40% of African Americans and Hispanics with type 2 diabetes do not consider heart disease and diabetes to be related conditions.

A Deadly Complication of Diabetes

In fact, heart disease is the leading cause of death among people with type 2 diabetes. African Americans and Hispanics are more than twice as likely to develop type 2 diabetes as compared with Caucasians.

Survey results also showed that nearly 50% of African Americans and Hispanics with type 2 diabetes do not understand the connection between heart disease and insulin resistance—a primary underlying cause of type 2 diabetes. Insulin resistance, considered an independent risk factor for cardiovascular disease, occurs when the body fails to respond properly to its own insulin. Certain ethnic populations, such as African Americans and Hispanics, are more insulin resistant than Caucasians, causing them to be at high risk for both type 2 diabetes and heart disease.

"Heart disease is the leading cause of death for African Americans and Hispanics, and the most deadly of the diabetes-related complications," said Elizabeth Ofili, MD, MPH, chief of cardiology, Morehouse

School of Medicine, Atlanta, Georgia, and ABC president. "The results of this survey sound an alarm that education is needed to ensure high-risk populations are aware of the strong link between diabetes and heart disease, and the need to take the necessary steps to prevent or manage these diseases over time."

African Americans and Hispanics are more likely to develop serious complications resulting from uncontrolled type 2 diabetes. The most effective way to measure how well a person's diabetes is being controlled over time is the A1c test, which provides a picture of blood sugar levels during a 3-month period. Although the A1c test is a key tool in the management of diabetes, nearly 40% of respondents with type 2 diabetes could not define the purpose of the test and 50% of the respondents with type 2 diabetes did not know what their target A1c level should be. Experts recommend a goal of 6.5–7.0% for optimal diabetes management.

"Inadequately treated diabetes, as indicated by higher than recommended A1c levels, is dangerous because of the potential risk of long-term complications. Research shows that for every percent above the A1c target level, a patient's risk of cardiovascular disease also increases," stated Samuel Dagogo-Jack, MD, FRCP, professor of medicine, Division of Endocrinology and Metabolism, University of Tennessee Health Science Center College of Medicine. "Tight control of diabetes is possible with diet, exercise and combination therapies, including drugs that target insulin resistance. These insulin sensitizers help patients use their own natural insulin more effectively."

Populations at Risk

The U.S. Centers for Disease Control and Prevention (CDC) has labeled diabetes "the epidemic of our time," with the greatest increase in certain ethnic populations. According to the U.S. Office of Minority Health, the prevalence of diabetes among African Americans is about 70% higher than in Caucasians and the prevalence in Hispanics is nearly double that of Caucasians. As of March 2002, it is estimated that 2.3 million African Americans and 1.2 million Hispanics have type 2 diabetes in the U.S. alone.

Despite ethnicity being a key risk factor in developing type 2 diabetes and its related complications such as heart disease, 50% of Hispanics and 48% of African Americans are not very or not at all concerned with developing type 2 diabetes. Similarly, 44% of Hispanics and 51% of African Americans are not very or not at all concerned with developing heart disease.

"Educating high-risk populations about the link between ethnicity, type 2 diabetes and heart disease is a critical step in managing this epidemic," stated B. Waine Kong, PhD, JD, chief executive officer, ABC. "The ABC urges everyone at high risk to talk to his or her doctor about ways to manage type 2 diabetes and help prevent complications."

THE PROBLEM OF DIABETIC EYE DISEASE

Jerry D. Cavallerano

In the following selection, optometrist Jerry D. Cavallerano describes one of the frightening complications of diabetes: diabetic retinopathy, damage to the retina of the eye. Unfortunately, diabetic retinopathy may develop without any symptoms or change in vision; for this reason, the author suggests, diabetics should receive regular eye exams. Blood glucose management has also proven to reduce the risks of diabetic retinopathy. According to Cavallerano, a combination of diligent glucose control, regular eye examinations, and high-tech surgery can reduce the risks of vision loss due to diabetic retinopathy. Cavallerano is assistant to the director of the Beetham Eye Institute of the Joslin Diabetes Center in Boston, Massachusetts.

Your eyes are delicate. Each one contains some of the smallest structures in your body, from the cornea, which is the clear "front window" that helps focus light into the eye, to the network of tiny blood vessels that supply the eyes with oxygen.

Unfortunately, your eyes, in their delicacy, are susceptible to the effects of diabetes. For example, fluctuations in blood glucose levels can affect your vision. Diabetes can prompt cataracts to develop earlier in life than they otherwise might, and diabetes is a risk factor for glaucoma.

The most significant effect of diabetes on the eye, however, is diabetic retinopathy. Diabetic retinopathy is the result of damage to the retina of the eye. The retina is the light-sensitive tissue that lines the inner surface of the eye. It receives focused light rays and transforms the light image into nerve signals that the brain interprets as vision.

The Scope of Diabetic Eye Disease

There are several different categories of diabetic retinopathy: Nonproliferative diabetic retinopathy, proliferative diabetic retinopathy, and diabetic macular edema.

In nonproliferative retinopathy, high blood glucose levels cause structural, functional, and hormonal changes in the retina that affect the retina's small blood vessels. Changes in blood vessel walls allow fluids to leak into the retinal tissue. Furthermore, changes in blood circulation result in less oxygen-rich blood circulating in the retina. These changes in blood vessels and circulation damage retinal tissue.

Proliferative retinopathy is more involved. In proliferative retinopathy, the retina releases chemical messengers that stimulate the growth of new blood vessels to bring more oxygen to the retina. Unfortunately, the new vessels leak fluids such as blood and blood products into the retina. They may even burst and fill the back of the eye with blood, causing significant vision loss. What's more, scar tissue accompanying the new vessels can pull on the retina, distorting vision and eventually detaching the retina from the underlying tissue. Retinal detachment can threaten your sight.

Leakage from diseased or abnormal retinal vessels may cause a sight-threatening build-up of fluid in the macula, the central area of the retina that allows you to see fine details clearly. Fluid build-up here is called macular edema.

The Symptoms

Diabetic retinopathy usually has no symptoms when it first starts to develop. It's even possible to have severe, sight-threatening retinopathy without having any change in vision. When symptoms do occur, they may include black or red "floaters," or spots, in your field of vision. Macular edema can blur or distort your vision, and straight lines may appear warped. Macular edema can also affect how you see colors.

Keep in mind that some changes in vision may be related to diabetes but not indicate diabetic retinopathy. For example, elevated blood glucose may make you near-sighted or far-sighted, and the near-sightedness and far-sightedness may come and go. Diabetes puts you at risk for cataracts, which cloud the lens and can make you feel as though you are looking through waxed paper. And some changes in vision may simply be a product of aging. If you're older than 50, changes in the fluid that fills the eyeball (the vitreous) can cause translucent or web-like floaters that move as your eye moves.

Diagnosing Diabetic Retinopathy

Because retinopathy can exist without any symptoms, *waiting for symptoms means waiting too long for treatment.* Comprehensive, regularly scheduled dilated eye examinations are the best way to diagnose diabetic retinopathy at a time when it is most amenable to treatment. A comprehensive eye exam entails more than looking at letters on a chart across the room. To detect retinopathy, your eye doctor must dilate your pupils with eyedrops and look at the inside of your eye. . . .

People with type 1 generally don't develop retinopathy before puberty, but once they are 10 years old, they should have an initial comprehensive eye exam 3 to 5 years after diagnosis with diabetes.

Once someone has had type 1 for 15 years, there is a higher likelihood of developing retinopathy; vision-threatening proliferative retinopathy is present in 25 percent of those who have had type 1 for more than 15 years.

People with type 2 are more likely to have retinopathy at the time of diabetes diagnosis or shortly thereafter. Therefore, they should get an eye exam as soon as possible after they are told they have diabetes.

Regardless of whether you have type 1 or type 2, once you've had an initial comprehensive eye exam, you should get one at least once a year, more often if you develop hypertension, kidney disease, or elevated cholesterol, or if your diabetes is poorly controlled.

Women contemplating pregnancy should have a comprehensive eye exam before getting pregnant, and pregnant women should have a comprehensive eye exam early in the first trimester, and at least once more during the pregnancy, depending on the recommendation of the eye doctor.

Treating Diabetic Eye Disease

There is no guaranteed way to prevent retinopathy or to cure it once it has set in. Fortunately, however, over the past 25 years, several treatments have emerged that can substantially reduce the risk of vision loss from retinopathy. The first is laser surgery. Laser surgery is generally recommended for people who have high-risk proliferative retinopathy or significant diabetic macular edema. There are two kinds of laser surgery: focal laser photocoagulation and scatter laser photocoagulation. These surgeries are performed by retinal specialists, who are ophthalmologists trained and experienced in treating diseases of the retina.

Focal laser photocoagulation is performed for diabetic macular edema. A person with clinically significant macular edema has about a 30 percent risk of moderate vision loss. For example, vision may decrease so that the person will be able to see 4 fewer lines of letters on the standard eye chart. Laser photocoagulation can reduce this risk to approximately 12 percent.

In focal laser photocoagulation, the retinal specialist uses fluorescein angiography photography to reveal specific areas in the retina that are leaking fluid into the macula. The specialist injects a dye into a vein in the person's arm, and the dye travels to the eyes. A special camera takes a series of photographs in rapid sequence to document the flow of dye through the vessels and highlight any vessels that are diseased or leaking. Then the retinal specialist focuses a brief burst of light on the leaking areas to seal them off.

Focal laser photocoagulation usually requires fewer than 100 applications of the laser. A follow-up examination is usually recommended 8 to 12 weeks after treatment.

Proliferative diabetic retinopathy poses a significant risk of severe vision loss. For example, people affected by proliferative diabetic retinopathy may lose so much of their vision they can see only the large "E" on most eye charts at a distance of five feet. The risk of severe vision loss from high-risk proliferative diabetic retinopathy over a year may be as high as 60 percent. Scatter laser photocoagulation reduces this risk to approximately 2 to 4 percent over a total of five years if the laser surgery is performed in a timely fashion.

In scatter laser photocoagulation, the retinal specialist does not treat the diseased areas directly. Rather, he or she focuses the laser on areas away from the center of the retina. Indirect treatment reduces the stimulus that causes new vessels to grow. Generally, scatter laser photocoagulation requires 1,200 to 1,800 applications spread over two or three treatment sessions. People who've had the treatment are usually requested to come back for a follow-up evaluation three months after the last treatment.

For those with both clinically significant macular edema and high-risk proliferative retinopathy, focal and scatter laser photocoagulation may be necessary.

Focal and scatter laser photocoagulation surgery are usually done in an ophthalmologist's office. The only anesthesia required is an eye-drop that is also routinely used for comprehensive dilated eye examinations. Your vision may be blurred for a few hours following laser photocoagulation because of the eyedrops.

It's important to remember that laser surgery does not cure diabetic retinopathy. The goal of laser surgery is to reduce the risk of vision loss. Possible side effects of laser photocoagulation include a smaller field of peripheral vision and difficulty with night vision. Peripheral vision is your outer, indirect field of vision—think of when you see something "out of the corner" of your eye.

Diabetic retinopathy may progress despite laser photocoagulation surgery. Burst or leaking blood vessels may still hemorrhage blood into the vitreous, or scar tissue may pull on the retina. In such cases, the ophthalmologist may perform a vitrectomy. During a vitrectomy, the ophthalmologist draws the vitreous out of the eyeball and replaces it with saline solution or another fluid. A vitrectomy must be performed in an operating room, and it usually requires a local anesthetic. The ophthalmologist may also perform laser surgery at the same time to further reduce the risk of recurrent bleeding from burst or leaking blood vessels.

Complete recovery may take up to three to six months, but most of the healing occurs within four weeks. Careful follow-up is necessary to monitor for new hemorrhages, infection, or increased eye pressure.

Lowering the Risk

There is no method guaranteed to completely prevent diabetic retinopathy. However, you can lower your risk of developing it by controlling your blood glucose. The Diabetes Control and Complications Trial (DCCT) and the United Kingdom Prospective Diabetes Study (UKPDS) both illustrate that intensive blood glucose control greatly reduces the risk of onset and progression of diabetic retinopathy. In the DCCT, people with type 1 who were on intensive therapy reduced diabetic retinopathy by 35 to 74 percent. They reduced the appearance of severe nonproliferative retinopathy and proliferative retinopathy, and the need for laser surgery, by 45 percent. They also reduced the first appearance of any retinopathy by 27 percent. The UKPDS found similar results for people with type 2.

Medical management of diabetes, regular follow-up eye examinations, and laser photocoagulation as necessary can significantly reduce the risk of vision loss from retinopathy. Two major clinical trials have demonstrated the value of laser surgery and one major clinical trial has shown the value of vitrectomy. Studies of new oral medications specifically for treating eye problems are under way. Researchers are also investigating ways to alter blood flow to prevent the early changes of diabetic retinopathy.

THE COMPLICATIONS OF DIABETIC NERVE DISEASE

Wayne L. Clark

According to Wayne L. Clark, diabetic neuropathy, nerve disease, is the most common complication of diabetes. In the following selection, Clark discusses the nature and progression of diabetic nerve disease, efforts to understand its causes, and strategies to manage its complications. Because all organs and systems of the body contain nerves, Clark explains, diabetic nerve disease can affect all parts of the body; as a result, diabetics may suffer from sexual dysfunction and bladder and stomach problems. One of the most debilitating complications, however, is sores on the feet that do not heal, which can ultimately lead to amputation. Managing blood glucose levels that are impaired by diabetes has been shown to decrease nerve disease, but the best treatment is early detection. Because diabetic nerve damage often results in a loss of sensation, many diabetics do not know there is a problem before it is too late. The author recommends that screening for nerve disease be part of every routine examination. Clark is a longtime contributor to *Countdown* magazine, a publication of the Juvenile Diabetes Foundation.

John McDonough lived with Type 1 diabetes for a long time before he had to devote much thought to diabetic neuropathy [nerve disease]. He was diagnosed at age 6, but it was over thirty years later that the most common complication of diabetes began to dramatically complicate his life.

"I started having perceived pain in my feet, especially at night," he says. "It would keep me from sleeping. It was particularly bad when my sugars were either high or low, or so it seemed."

At that time, in his early 40s, McDonough was an energetic and successful businessman. At 63, while chief executive officer of Newell Rubbermaid, Inc., McDonough turned his struggle with Type 1 diabetes into a fight for the cure, as the chairman of the Juvenile Diabetes Foundation International (JDF). All of his efforts to fight dia-

From "When Diabetes Strikes a Nerve," by Wayne L. Clark, *Countdown*, Spring 2000. Copyright © 2000 by Juvenile Diabetes Foundation International. Reprinted with permission.

betes didn't stop the complications of his own disease, however, and in 1998, he lost his left leg to diabetic neuropathy.

"It started as a small sore on my toe that wouldn't heal," he says. "We couldn't do anything with it. Then it became infected, then we decided to amputate one toe, then the next, and finally the leg."

Unfortunately, John McDonough isn't unique in this respect. Diabetes is the leading cause of amputations other than those from accidents. Diabetic neuropathy, combined with damage to small blood vessels, is the culprit.

As researchers learn more and more about the mechanisms involved in diabetic neuropathy, they are developing new tools and innovative strategies to aid in the early detection and treatment of the disease. In February 2000, the JDF Center for Complications of Diabetes at the University of Michigan in Ann Arbor had its formal introduction. This $6.6-million center is designed to develop methods for preventing the destructive processes that lead to both diabetic neuropathy and diabetic retinopathy (eye disease), as well as to develop effective therapies for treating both complications.

A Slow, Silent Process

It was pain in his feet that sent John McDonough to his doctor, but the process that led up to it had been going on silently for many years. The culprit, as with most complications of diabetes, is elevated blood glucose. A complex and not clearly understood cascade of cellular events, fed by the presence of too much sugar, leads to a "dying back" of the nerve fibers.

"Think of a nerve as an electrical cord," says Eva Feldman, M.D., Ph.D., University of Michigan neurologist and associate director of the JDF Center for Complications of Diabetes. "The nerve fiber itself is the wire inside the cord, and it is surrounded by insulation. In diabetic neuropathy, the nerve fiber itself becomes damaged at its farthest points, and the insulation also becomes damaged. Also, the cell body that supplies the nerve becomes dysfunctional and dies."

Not only do the nerves die back from the ends, but the longest nerves—those that go to the toes, for instance, which are the longest peripheral nerves—are affected first. The destruction of the myelin sheath that insulates them causes further dysfunction, like a short-circuit in a wire with broken insulation. The final insult of neuropathy is the death of the cells that supply the nerve with food and fuel.

Smaller nerve fibers are affected first, and their dying back reduces pain and temperature sensation. The loss of the larger nerves, responsible for sensing vibration and for the reflexes, compound the sensory deficits.

Diabetic neuropathy is an inclusive term for a number of syndromes that can affect people with diabetes. Estimates vary, but it is thought that 60 percent or more of people with diabetes have some degree of neuropathy. It can develop within ten years of the onset of the disease, and affects people with both Type 1 and Type 2 diabetes. It is exacerbated by poor glucose control, and by smoking.

The most common form is peripheral diabetic polyneuropathy, the kind that John McDonough experienced. This type of neuropathy is responsible for the seemingly paradoxical symptoms reported by many people with diabetes: lack of sensation or numbness, and burning or stabbing pain. It can affect the feet, legs, arms, and hands.

"I describe it to my patients as Alzheimer's disease of the peripheral nerves," says Douglas A. Greene, M.D., director of the JDF Center for Complications of Diabetes, and chief of endocrinology and metabolism at the University of Michigan Medical Center. "It is a degeneration of the nerves, and is a dynamic process in which degeneration and regeneration are occurring simultaneously. The net balance between these two processes determines whether the neuropathy progresses, regresses, or stabilizes."

Autonomic neuropathy is a serious disorder that, according to one estimate, may already affect a quarter of all people with diabetes at the time of their diagnosis, particularly people with Type 2 diabetes. It may affect the digestive system, the sexual organs, the urinary tract, the heart, and even the sweat glands. Symptoms come in a wide variety of forms, including sexual dysfunction, delayed emptying of the stomach, diarrhea, and bladder abnormalities.

"We think that autonomic neuropathy may be an important factor in excess cardiovascular mortality in people with diabetes," Dr. Greene says. "Diabetic patients often show up with congestive heart failure even though they don't have a history of heart attacks. That's because they've had 'silent' heart attacks because they don't feel cardiac pain."

A third form, focal neuropathies, may affect the eyes, facial muscles, hearing, penis and lower back, thighs, or abdomen. As the name implies, they are focused on very specific nerves or areas. The effects are often described as twinges, jabbing pains, twitches, or palsies.

The Blood Sugar Connection

The dysfunction and death of the nerves in neuropathy is well understood, but why and how it happens is not yet known. Generally, it is thought that there are three contributing processes: metabolic, vascular, and neurodegenerative. Further, according to Dr. Greene, there is one overarching theme to all three of these: oxidative stress. High glucose levels produce a series of interrelated changes in the metabolism of proteins and lipids in cells of the nerves and eyes that lead to the generation of oxygen free radicals, highly reactive molecules that are toxic and can cause injury to healthy cells and tissues.

"This state of oxidative stress further impairs sick nerve and eye cells by depleting their supply of blood and growth factors, which leads to a type of cell death known as apoptosis," explains Dr. Greene. "Unchecked, oxidative stress and resulting apoptosis lead to loss of nerve and eye function and the resulting diabetic complications of neuropathy and retinopathy."

Excess glucose can lead to oxidative stress by two major processes, known as non-enzymatic glycation and the aldose reductase pathway. Both processes create oxidative free radicals through parallel mechanisms, setting in motion a cascade of harmful cellular events that is collectively called "oxidative stress." Oxidative stress damages the nerve cells directly, and also damages the blood vessels that supply them. Damaged blood vessels fail to deliver blood, and this "ischemia" further accelerates oxidative stress. To make matters worse, intermittent ischemia, where the blood supply is interrupted and then restored, is one of the greatest creators of oxygen free radicals.

This vicious cycle of metabolic crises is fueled by sugar, and control of blood sugar is the first line of defense against it. The Diabetes Complications and Control Trial demonstrated conclusively that there was at least a 60 percent decrease in neuropathy with improved control. In fact, good control of blood sugar levels using insulin—or oral agents, drugs used to control blood sugar levels in patients with Type 2 diabetes—can not only delay the onset of neuropathy, but can reportedly improve symptoms for those already affected.

A New Line of Defense

Other drugs that might stop the oxidative stress or its consequences are under investigation. For instance, neurotrophic factors, among the newest potential therapies for neuropathy, are proteins that promote the survival of nerve tissue and may also promote its regeneration. The action of neurotrophins was first described half a century ago, but only in the past few years have some types been tested in clinical trials of neuropathy treatment. The results have been encouraging, and more trials both alone and in combination are in the offing.

Since neuropathy is a multifactorial disease, a multifactorial treatment seems to make sense and is at the forefront of research efforts under way at the JDF Center for Complications of Diabetes.

"We feel combination therapy is the watchword," Dr. Greene says, "since no existing therapy completely corrects any of the three components. We're combining metabolic treatment with antioxidants and neurotrophic factors. The use of vasodilators is also important, to help keep the blood flow to the cells."

Drs. Greene and Feldman, and their colleagues at the University of Michigan, hope to prove the basic science of the combination approach to therapy. They hope to demonstrate that neuropathy can be stabilized, reduced, or even prevented by:

- blood sugar control to limit the cause of the process;
- aldose reductase inhibitors to interrupt the metabolic disarray;

- antioxidants to fight the destruction caused by oxidative free radicals;
- and neurotrophic factors to encourage the regeneration of nerve tissue.

Then, the researchers can begin a clinical trial in humans.

Better Treatment for Painful Symptoms

Meanwhile, there is symptomatic help available now for those who have painful neuropathy. Some antiepileptic drugs, such as gabapentin and carbamazepine, as well as certain tricyclic antidepressants, such as amitriptyline and nortriptyline, have been shown to be effective in reducing extreme pain associated with diabetic neuropathy. Capsaicin creams, applied topically, also provide relief for some people.

Pain management, oddly enough, may be needed by some people even as their neuropathy improves. Dr. Greene points out that an increase in pain as blood sugar control is improved is actually a good sign. The seeming paradox may be due to improved nerve health allowing the person to feel pain they simply couldn't feel before, or to the "misfiring" of nerves as they make new connections.

Symptomatic treatments are also available for various autonomic neuropathies. Viagra is helpful in treating erectile dysfunction, and cisapride and metoclopramide are used for treating gastrointestinal problems. Autonomic neuropathy can also produce unexpected drops in blood pressure on standing, and unexplained rapid heartbeat; and medications can help with both.

Early Intervention Is Vital

Early detection and intervention will become increasingly important as new treatments become available. The earlier therapy is started, the greater the likelihood of saving and regenerating nerve tissue. The problem is the early signs and symptoms of diabetic neuropathy are often overlooked. It has been said that many or even most people with diabetic neuropathy do not have symptoms, and to some extent this might be true. But Dr. Greene says that the issue might be how carefully one looks for the symptoms.

"The major risks of neuropathy are through deficits," Dr. Greene says. "For instance, the foot most likely to ulcerate and be amputated is not the foot of a person experiencing lots of painful symptoms— rather, it's the foot of someone who has no sensation at all.

"If a patient has painful feet, he or she will come in and say 'I really hurt.' That patient may have mild neuropathy. The patient with advanced neuropathy very likely has symptoms, but is not aware of what to attribute them to. It may be poor balance, inability to walk long distances, recurrent foot sores, difficulty with fine coordination such as buttoning a shirt. Until the patient sits down and talks to a physician who does a complete history, these symptoms may not be seen as symptoms of the disease, because they're subtle and not likely to lead to independent complaints.

"Part of the reason it's not high on the radar screens of patients and physicians," Dr. Greene continues, "is that there's no treatment yet. Diseases for which there is no agreed-upon therapy are often diseases where signs and symptoms are not actively sought."

There are a growing number of tools to help diagnose diabetic neuropathy and measure its severity, but as a practical matter they are primarily of interest to clinicians and researchers. There are nerve conduction studies, blood studies, cerebrospinal fluid analyses, nerve and muscle biopsies, and other methods of getting a detailed picture of nerve damage. But there are simple, noninvasive ways to screen the average patient for neuropathy, and they should be part of every routine examination.

Type 2 Diabetes and Neuropathy

New knowledge about who is at risk for developing Type 2 diabetes may help people become aware of their risk for neuropathy earlier. One reason is that the definition of Type 2 diabetes itself is being challenged, as the line between impaired glucose tolerance (IGT) and Type 2 diabetes becomes less clear. Currently, IGT describes a condition in which a person's blood sugar level is higher than normal, but not high enough to qualify as diabetes. It is a common precursor to Type 2 diabetes.

"It may be that people with impaired glucose tolerance have an increased prevalence of neuropathy," Dr. Greene says. "Damage to the eyes has been the traditional benchmark for damage from diabetes, but it may be that peripheral nerves are even more sensitive to minor abnormalities in glucose levels. We may need to actually redefine diabetes based on the most sensitive endorgan. It's an interesting semantic argument that is just beginning to emerge."

What this means for people with Type 2 diabetes or at risk for Type 2 diabetes is that vigilance and early detection are critical. "New guidelines lower the threshold for defining impaired glucose tolerance," Dr. Feldman says. "We recently published a study in collaboration with other centers in which we found that in our patient population, when someone is sent to us with numb, aching feet of unknown cause, one-third have IGT. So early diagnosis is key, and I believe that IGT is the first step toward Type 2 diabetes and that we need early diagnosis and treatment for signs of neuropathy."

Success Will Be Far-Reaching

Progress in treating and preventing diabetic neuropathy may ultimately help people with other neurodegenerative diseases, as well. First, there are neuropathies that are caused by other syndromes; and there is also an age-related, spontaneously occurring idiopathic neuropathy. Then there are other, often devastating degenerative diseases of both the peripheral and central nervous system.

"There's an underlying common thread in nerve damage," Dr. Feldman says, "whether it's in the brain—such as in Alzheimer's disease, Parkinson's disease, and Huntington's—or in the peripheral nerves. In all these disorders, it appears that cells undergo a similar process of programmed cell death. It's likely due at least in part to oxidative stress. So if we understand and clearly treat one neurodegenerative disease, such as diabetic neuropathy, there should be clear applicability to other neurodegenerative disorders. As a neurologist, I'm pretty excited about that."

John McDonough is still working hard despite his health problems, leading a $17-billion corporation and leading JDF toward a cure. For his own part, he's now on an insulin pump, which has improved his control. The symptoms in his right foot have improved, especially the pain at night that kept him from sleeping. What he'd really like is to make the pain of diabetes better for everyone.

"My paternal grandfather died of the complications of diabetes in the late 1920s, just about the time insulin was becoming available," he says. "Our oldest daughter is 41 years old, and has been insulin-dependent for 17 years. I also have five other children, and five grandchildren. We really don't want to see any more of this disease. I'd like to be the guy who hosts the 'going out of business' party for JDF."

As research efforts like those under way at the JDF Center for Complications of Diabetes progress, John McDonough is certain to see significant progress toward solving the remaining mysteries of diabetic neuropathy and its devastating attack on the nervous system.

THE HIGH PREVALENCE OF AMPUTATION IN DIABETIC MINORITIES

Carol S. Saunders

Research shows a higher rate of lower extremity amputations (LEAs) among diabetic minorities, writes Carol S. Saunders in the following selection. Saunders points out that this disparity may not be due to physical differences, but to differences in access to health care. For example, Saunders explains, social, cultural, and economic factors such as lack of health insurance make it difficult for minorities to get proper treatment. The biggest problem, Saunders reveals, is poor foot care; foot injuries or trauma from inappropriate shoes are the most common triggers for the foot ulcers that lead to LEAs. Saunders describes the physiological conditions that contribute to the nerve disease that leads to LEAs and explains how difficult it is for patients to recognize the symptoms. However, according to Saunders, studies also show that screening, education, and aggressive treatment have been effective in reducing amputation rates among minorities. Saunders is senior editor of *Patient Care*, a magazine for health professionals that focuses on diagnosis, treatment, and prevention.

Although lower extremity amputations are performed more often in minority patients than in whites, the reasons are probably related to access to care and sociocultural issues, not metabolic factors. Simple, effective interventions can reduce amputation rates by up to 85%.

The cascade leading to lower extremity amputation (LEA) starts with the development of the inevitable scourge of diabetes—neuropathy [nerve disease]. The resulting reduced sensation in the feet, when combined with an acute or repetitive trauma, leads to a foot ulcer. Because blood flow to the feet may be reduced by peripheral vascular disease, another diabetes complication, the ulcer may not heal and becomes infected. Chronic ulceration occurs, which in turn leads to ischemia [constriction or obstruction of the blood vessels] and gangrene and the need for LEA.

Any LEA is a crisis that probably could have been prevented and

Excerpted from "Preventing Amputation in Patients with Diabetes," by Carol S. Saunders, *Patient Care*, May 15, 2000. Copyright © 2000 by Medical Economics Company, Inc. Reprinted with permission.

thus represents a failure of the patient's self-care and also of the health care system. Compounding this failure is the fact that so many more minority patients than whites receive LEA instead of preventive or conservative care. Proven, simple interventions at many different stages of the cascade can prevent the loss of a toe, foot, or limb, but these strategies must be implemented on a widespread basis to be effective. While improved nutrition and glycemic [blood glucose] control are certainly important, they are not the main tools in the path to preventing amputation. Screening of minority patients at risk and implementing proper foot care are the most critical components, and patient education plays a large role.

The Scope of the Problem

Why do blacks and other minorities have higher rates of LEAs compared to whites? No known clinical reason accounts for why the rates are higher, and most experts agree that lack of access to care and other social barriers largely explain the difference. This suggests that if all patients were provided with the same opportunities for care, amputation rates in minority and white patients would probably be similar.

Social issues that may impede care include language barriers or illiteracy. In rural areas, the physical distance to travel to a physician may be too great to be practical. In urban areas, medical and transportation costs may be high. Although much data has been gathered on the prevalence of LEA in minority patients, the unique sociocultural characteristics of specific minority groups that may lead to higher risk factors for LEA have not yet been studied.

Reduction and even elimination of the racial disparity in LEAs [was] a major focus of the Healthy People 2000 program, continues as a primary focus of the Healthy People 2010 program, and can be a priority in the practice of primary care. According to a statement from the US Department of Health and Human Services, one goal of the Healthy People program is to "reduce lower extremity amputation rates from diabetes among blacks by 40% from their 1995 levels."

The Prevalence of Amputation

In what is considered the longest prospective study (more than 20 years) of the effects of race and diabetes on the risk of LEA in 14,407 subjects, it was shown that the rate of LEAs was 2.8 times higher in blacks than in whites. Multivariate analyses indicated, however, that race did not play as large a role when environment, education, smoking, and hypertension were considered. When adjusted for these factors, the race difference became insignificant. Indeed, an additional association was found between socioeconomic status and risk of LEA among white subjects, supporting the theory that it is access to health care and not some metabolic or racial factor causing the different rates.

Other studies show similar findings. One sought to identify the incidence of LEAs in minorities in south Texas in order to implement the goals in the Healthy People 2000 program. Of the 1,043 patients with an LEA studied in 1993, 815 were Mexican American, 71 were black, and 157 were non-Hispanic whites. While the authors of this study hypothesize that cultural issues may be involved in the higher minority rates (such as patient reliance on folk healing or alternative remedies instead of allopathic [traditional] medical care), they ultimately conclude that culturally sensitive patient education would lead to a substantial reduction in LEA rates.

An additional disparity exists in postoperative care because mortality rates after LEA are higher in minority patients. Although sex and level of amputation also affect mortality (with women having higher rates), one study found that race affected mortality rates when 8,169 hospitalizations for LEA in California in 1991 were studied. Age-adjusted mortality rates per 1,000 amputations were 41.39 for blacks, 19.69 for Hispanics, and 34.98 for non-Hispanic whites. As in the other studies, these authors suggest that lack of health insurance plays a large role in the rate differences.

In addition to being inordinately high in minority patients, rates of LEAs are exceedingly high across the general population. Because hospitals keep detailed records on major operations such as LEAs, plentiful data are available. According to the American Diabetes Association, more than 50,000 LEAs are performed each year in patients with diabetes. In 1996, the number was 54,000, a 29% increase over 1980. A small decline in amputation rates between 1983 and 1992 is attributed to reduced prevalence of smoking, hypertension, and heart disease—but not diabetes.

Foot ulcers are the cause of 85% of all LEAs. They account for more than 162,000 hospitalizations annually, and patients with diabetes account for 46% of these. A foot ulcer will develop in 15% of all people with diabetes in their lifetime. Only about 3% of the population have diabetes, but this population accounts for over 50% of all nontraumatic LEAs.

Amidst all the disturbing statistics, one encouraging fact stands out—that interventions to prevent LEAs are effective, and they work well in minority patients. For example, in a study of an amputation prevention program in primary care, a "remarkable" 48% reduction in amputation rates in 639 Native American patients with diabetes was achieved when aggressive care was provided. The study reviewed 3 periods of care: a 4-year period in which care at the discretion of the provider was given; a 4-year period in which screening for foot problems and foot care education was offered; and a 3-year period in which a comprehensive program was implemented that included glycemic control and a systemized, algorithmic approach to foot care. In the standard care period, the annual LEA incidence was 29 per 1,000 diabetic-person years. The incidence in the screening and education period was 21 per 1,000 diabetic-person years but was only 15 for the systemized period.

The Risk Factors

People who eventually need LEA do not necessarily have poor glycemic control, although this is usually a contributing factor. Poor foot care is more likely to have a direct effect on LEA rates. Either acute trauma from an injury or repetitive trauma from mechanical pressure from a foot deformity or inappropriate shoes is the trigger for most ulcers that lead to amputation. The presence of peripheral neuropathy and/or peripheral vascular disease increases the risk as well.

The risk factors for LEAs are virtually the same as those for foot ulcers in people with either type 1 or type 2 diabetes. The risk of foot ulcers and amputation increase 2- to 4-fold with age and duration of diabetes, according to the authors of a position statement from the American Diabetes Association entitled "Preventive Foot Care in People With Diabetes." Older people have higher rates of ulceration because the diabetic complications of neuropathy and peripheral vascular disease take years to do their damage.

At low risk are patients who do not have peripheral neuropathy and whose pedal [foot] pulses are present. Patients with no severe deformities, no ulcers, and no prior amputations are also low risk.

Smoking increases risk, as do high alcohol consumption, comorbid [coexisting] conditions, and lack of patient knowledge of preventive foot care. Men have a higher risk, but the reasons for this are not yet known. A foot problem still leads to a diagnosis of diabetes far too often, suggesting that too-late diagnosis of diabetes is a risk factor as well. Rarely does one risk factor itself precipitate LEA; a combination is usually present, such as an ulcer plus a comorbid condition including peripheral neuropathy or peripheral vascular disease.

The most important intervention to prevent amputation that can be performed in primary care is screening to identify patients at risk for diabetic foot ulcers. The loss of sensation associated with diabetic peripheral neuropathy has been clearly shown to provide an environment in which ulcers easily develop. All patients with diabetes need to have their feet examined at every office visit. . . .

The Conditions That Lead to Amputation

The longer the duration of diabetes, the higher the risk for microvascular and macrovascular complications of diabetes, specifically peripheral neuropathy and peripheral vascular disease. These are the main conditions that lead to the development of foot ulceration and thus amputation.

Distal symmetric sensorimotor polyneuropathy [nerve damage in the extremities that impairs sensation] affects nearly 50% of patients who have had diabetes for more than 15 years and increases the risk of ulcer and/or amputation by 20%. As soon as diabetes develops, so does neuropathy. Even before clinically significant neuropathy is manifested, electrodiagnostic testing of the nerves detects changes because the peripheral nerves are very sensitive to alterations in blood glucose levels.

Neuropathy develops slowly over the years and is not reversible. The symptoms change and may not be the same throughout the day or from week to week. Symptoms include sensory alteration, including pain, numbness, or tingling in the feet, but most patients are not aware of the most common sign—loss of sensation—which exacerbates any foot problem.

Neuropathy also leads to motor abnormalities by causing atrophy of the intrinsic muscles, allowing the foot to take abnormal form and position. Prominent metatarsal heads develop, causing additional pressure on the foot that leads to altered posture and gait, and ultimately, ulceration.

A reduction in the blood supply to the small nerves in distal areas negatively affects oxygenation and delivery of nutrients. Signs include an absent pulse and arterial calcification. The resulting condition does not cause ulcers or amputations per se, but because the condition delays wound healing and hastens gangrene, it is a major part of the amputation cascade. The condition can develop in the general population but is 2 to 3 times more likely in those with diabetes.

Symptoms include intermittent claudication or rest pain that is relieved by changing position. These pain sensations may be hard to detect by a patient who also has peripheral neuropathy, and clinical examination is inexact. Signs of peripheral vascular disease that are not as significant as lack of palpable pulses but are still important are loss of foot hair, dependent rubor [redness], and coolness of the skin of the foot.

Although angiography [examination of the blood vessels] is the gold standard for diagnosis of peripheral vascular disease, it should only be used if vascular surgery is being considered. The ankle-arm index (AAI) or ankle-brachial index is more practical for office use and involves the ratio of blood pressure (BP) of the arm to BP of the leg. An AAI of less than 0.9 is considered positive for peripheral vascular disease.

Exercise may improve the condition, as will stopping smoking. Revascularization is possible but usually not practical or helpful.

If an ulcer or other foot wound is detected, treatment should be implemented immediately. When executed properly, treatment is extremely efficacious. For example, at a clinic designed for preventing LEA in people with diabetic foot ulcers, 87% of the 124 observed patients did not need amputation after primary ulceration after 3 years.

THE DIABETIC EMPLOYEE AND THE AMERICANS WITH DISABILITIES ACT

Mary B. Dickson

According to Mary B. Dickson, most diabetics need no special treatment by employers; in fact, those diabetics who manage their disease are extremely self-disciplined and responsible. Unfortunately, the author observes, fear and misunderstanding of diabetes may lead to discrimination. In the following selection, the author discusses what employers can do to provide reasonable accommodations for diabetic employees and comply with the Americans with Disabilities Act. Diabetes is a very individualized condition, the author writes, and most diabetics have few restrictions. Dickson explains that employers should balance the job's requirements and the individual's qualifications against each applicant's treatment regimen and the diabetic complications each experiences. While most need little if any accommodation, the author asserts, those with diabetic eye disease, for example, might require vision aids such as magnification and large-print documents. If these accommodations are viewed as "productivity enhancements," employers can get the most out of their diabetic employees. Dickson is president of Creative Compliance Management, a human resource consulting and training firm and author of *Supervising Employees with Disabilities: Beyond ADA Compliance*.

Diabetes mellitus results from the body's inability to use food effectively for energy, resulting in elevated blood sugar levels. Either the pancreas does not produce adequate insulin or the body cannot use the insulin effectively. There are two kinds of diabetes:

- Type I, appropriately called insulin-dependent diabetes (formerly called juvenile onset); OR
- Type II, known as non-insulin-dependent (formerly called adult onset diabetes). The title is not entirely accurate, since some Type II persons with diabetes must take insulin injections.

From "Employment Considerations for People Who Have Diabetes," by Mary B. Dickson, Program on Employment and Disability, School of Industrial and Labor Relations–Extension Division, Cornell University, December 18, 1997. Copyright © 1997 by Program on Employment and Disability. Reprinted with permission.

Type I diabetes represents only 5 to 10% of the 13,000,000 Americans with diabetes and is considered the more serious type. Once diagnosed, persons with diabetes Type I must monitor their blood sugar daily.

Persons with diabetes Type II, representing the other 90 to 95% of those with the condition, can control the disease with weight control, appropriate diet, and exercise. Many, but not all, take oral medication.

Half the people with diabetes do not know they have the condition. This may be dangerous since diabetes can lead to complications such as kidney problems, decreased vision, and foot disease, particularly if not well controlled. Employers may offer diabetes detection and education programs, using the resources of the local American Diabetes Association. This can alert employees to the symptoms of diabetes and encourage them to be tested so they can control the disease appropriately.

Diabetes cannot be cured, but it can be controlled. The person with diabetes needs to take responsibility for maintaining a good diet, exercising, and seeking appropriate medical care. Those who take good care of themselves can be healthier than other employees simply because they are knowledgeable about and participate in a healthy life-style.

Diabetes and the Americans with Disabilities Act

The Americans with Disabilities Act (ADA) defines disability in several ways, one of which is, "Someone who is regarded as having an impairment." Diabetes is not well known or understood by many employers. Many people with diabetes live and work successfully for years without negative impact on their work. Because their condition does not impact their ability to do their job, they may choose to not make their employer aware of their condition. Fear of discrimination keeps many employees with diabetes quiet. In what areas might employers discriminate? As with any disability, the potential to discriminate exists at any point in the employment process.

- A nurse sent her resume to 16 institutions, and in her cover letter mentioned her diabetes. She had only two responses, and no job offer.
- A man with diabetes initially hired to run a shipboard boutique was rejected by the company doctor because a diabetic woman passenger slipped into a coma 20 years ago and died, setting a precedent.
- An airline employee was forced to take two 10-minute breaks rather than one 20-minute break, during which time she had to test her blood sugar, take insulin, and eat. The change in her break schedule was insufficient time to complete the tasks required to maintain good diabetic control.

These situations reflect the fear and misunderstanding surrounding this condition. As with any other disability, employers are required by ADA to look at the actual limitations, not perceived limitations.

The Implications of Diabetes in the Workplace

Despite good monitoring of diet, medication, and exercise, some people with diabetes may experience insulin reactions caused by hypoglycemia (low blood sugar). Insulin reaction can be caused by not eating at appropriate times, irregular working schedules, and/or change in exercise level.

A person experiencing hypoglycemia may become suddenly weak, shaky, or faint. Many people with diabetes recognize these symptoms and will immediately drink orange juice or eat something high in sugar. It only takes a few minutes for the person's blood sugar to return to normal.

The American Diabetes Association states, "Diabetes as such should not be a cause for discriminating against any person in employment. People with diabetes should be individually considered for employment weighing such factors as the requirements or hazards of the specific job, the individual's medical condition, and their treatment regimen (diet, oral hypoglycemic agents, and insulin). Any person with diabetes, whether insulin-dependent or non-insulin-dependent, should be eligible for any employment for which he or she is otherwise qualified."

What Types of Jobs Do People with Diabetes Do?

There are very few restrictions for people with well controlled diabetes. Some laws prohibit people with insulin-treated diabetes from serving in the armed services and in jobs involving interstate driving and as pilots. Local laws may prohibit people with diabetes from serving on a police force. This continues to be a problem and the American Diabetes Association recommends each situation be considered on a case by case basis, even though a lawsuit was filed against the Maryland–National Capitol Park Police after which an officer with diabetes was reinstated. Problems may occur with those who cannot maintain blood sugar control, and consequently they should not work in dangerous areas. However, since this is quite uncommon, the employee, based on his or her experiences, should generally make this decision, not the employer. Diabetes is a highly individualized condition. Ideally, the employee, his or her doctor, and the employer work together to ensure success.

For the most part, people with diabetes should need no special treatment from their supervisors. An understanding of the condition and the possible need for regular work schedules and meal breaks is usually helpful and appreciated. Living successfully with diabetes means that a person must be self-disciplined, self-aware, and self-responsible, all valued characteristics in many jobs.

Enhancing Productivity on the Job

The Americans with Disabilities Act requires employers to "reasonably accommodate" the limitations imposed by a person's physical or mental disability. Reasonable accommodation is defined as modification or adjustment of a job, employment practice, or the work environment that makes it possible for a qualified person with a disability to be employed. The law states that the employer needs to accommodate from the first contact with the person with the disability, during the application process, on the job, in training, on the worksite, and when considering promotions and layoffs. If job duties change, new accommodations may need to be made. The ADA requires an employer to accommodate unless doing so would cause the employer an undue hardship.

If we think of accommodations as "productivity enhancements" similar to others made in the workplace, they become part of the cost of doing business. If that cost is an undue burden, however, the employer may offer the person with the disability an opportunity to provide the accommodation or assist in finding resources to pay for it. The ADA requires that employers only accommodate known disabilities. Some people with diabetes do experience complications such as vision loss. Visual impairment due to diabetes may be quite gradual, and the vision may fluctuate from day to day.

If the diabetes has resulted in visual loss, accommodations can be made. Low vision aids may prove useful. The employee's eye care professional may suggest magnification, appropriate lighting, or large print materials. The employee may want to contact a local resource center for people who are blind or visually impaired for a low vision assessment on the job to find useful aids. In some cases of diabetes, despite one's best efforts at maintaining good blood sugar control, the condition will progress. One's vision loss may be great enough that the person will need to learn alternative ways of performing activities. The employee may need to take a leave of absence to attend a formal program of vocational rehabilitation, where he or she will learn new ways to perform job duties. Vocational rehabilitation training will teach the person how to get around safely (perhaps with a white cane), use adaptive equipment, and perhaps perform job tasks in a somewhat different manner.

For most people with diabetes, the employer should have no concerns about training and promotion. If the employee's diabetes has caused significant functional limitations, and if training activities are planned, consult the employee about possible accommodations needed in the training environment.

These may include:
- regular testing of blood glucose levels and meal breaks
- training materials put into alternative formats such as large print

- having another trainee copy his or her notes if training is conducted in a darkened room

Employers should assume that people with diabetes have the same career goals and aspirations as any other employee. A person's diabetes should play no part in decisions about transfers and promotions. Concentrate only on the appropriateness of the person's skills for a new position and determine if reasonable accommodations are needed. Capitalize on the person's strengths and accommodate limitations to gain greatest productivity from the employee.

CHAPTER 2

THE CAUSES OF DIABETES

FACTORS THAT CONTRIBUTE TO THE ONSET OF DIABETES: AN OVERVIEW

Rattan Juneja, interviewed by Patrick Perry

In the following interview with Patrick Perry of the *Saturday Evening Post*, Rattan Juneja explains that a genetic predisposition alone is not the cause of diabetes; environmental factors such as diet and exercise play a significant role in the onset of the disease. For example, one theory suggests that some minority populations carry a "thrifty gene" that protects them during times of famine. However, Juneja reveals, when these populations adopt a Western lifestyle and become obese, an environmental factor that contributes to diabetes, they have a higher incidence of the disease. Because diabetes is a complex disease with many contributing factors, authorities recommend early screening for minorities and regular exams for anyone over forty. Juneja is a professor at the Indiana University School of Medicine in Bloomington and medical director of the Indiana Diabetes Center.

Patrick Perry: Experts estimate that 50 percent of Type 2 diabetics are undiagnosed in this country. How can so many diabetics go undetected? Are the symptoms of diabetes that subtle?

Rattan Juneja: In many cases of Type 2 diabetes, the diagnosis is made as an incidental finding. For example, you go to your doctor and for some reason, blood tests are drawn and a person might be found to have a blood sugar that is above the norm.

Diagnosing Two Different Diseases

Type 1 diabetics have a total and complete lack of insulin. But the brain needs a source of energy and utilizes glucose, which is broken down by insulin as the source of energy. The only other source of energy for the brain is through the breakdown of fats, which produces a condition called ketoacidosis—a condition that would make them very sick. People with ketoacidosis would be nauseous, vomiting, and very physically ill, which would bring them to the hospital. Type 1 diabetics often present with ketoacidosis, and then the diagnosis of diabetes is made.

Type 2 diabetes is a more complex disease. These people do produce insulin, but the insulin doesn't do what it is supposed to do. They have a condition of what we call insulin resistance where they are keeping their blood sugars at a certain level, and the insulin is still able to produce the energy needed, so the brain doesn't demand alternative sources of energy. There is no breakdown of fats due to lack of insulin. If anything, their insulin levels are higher than normal people's, so the condition goes undiagnosed for a long time until the glucose reaches a high threshold. Patients may not complain of increased thirst or increased urination. If you ever wore glasses when you were young, for example, every time your vision changed, you wouldn't realize it because you became used to seeing poorly. Undiagnosed diabetics get used to having blood sugars at a certain level, and this can go on for years.

In 1997, some experts urged earlier testing for diabetes, beginning at age 25. Is this recommendation still in effect? And if symptoms are so subtle, who should be tested early?

The March 2000 issue of *Diabetes Care* carried a consensus guideline statement from the American Diabetes Association (ADA). They are recommending testing for diabetes in high-risk populations every two years from age ten. Why would they come up with this kind of recommendation? The populations at high risk for Type 2 diabetes are non-Caucasian—African-Americans, Hispanics, Asians/South Pacific Islanders, American Indians, and Japanese-Americans.

The Thrifty Genes

In 1962, geneticist James Neel from the University of Michigan came up with the interesting hypothesis that people from certain ethnic minorities carry what he called the "thrifty gene." The highest incidence and prevalence of Type 2 diabetes occurs in the Pima Indians from Arizona. Almost 50 percent of Pima Indians will get Type 2 diabetes during their lifetimes. Why? If you look at the Pima Indians hundreds of years ago in their native environment, they belonged to a class of people that we would call the typical hunter-gatherer. Their lifestyle was basically hunting and subsistence farming. They were very, very active. But in subsistence farming, there were periods of famine. During those periods of famine, many people died. The Pima Indians who survived are thought to have carried genes that allowed them to conserve energy. We don't know what the gene is. We know that diabetes in most cases is a polygenic disorder; multiple genes are involved. Today, Native Americans, Indians, African-Americans, Asian Indians, and Japanese-Americans are potentially carrying that thrifty gene. I am an Asian Indian. If you take people with that thrifty gene and put us in an environment of plenty in the Western world—lack of activity, sitting in front of the computer or watching television, drinking high-calorie beverages, and going to fast-food restaurants—what happens to us? Because of that thrifty gene, we put on weight. And we know that obesity is related to insulin resistance. It becomes a vicious circle. You put on weight, develop insulin resistance, and then get diabetes.

There is another interesting theory called the thrifty phenotype. This theory relates to the fact that if you are born small, it may predispose you to getting Type 2 diabetes as you get older. This begs the question: Are minority kids smaller at birth as compared to Caucasian children? A large study looked at about four million birth weights of children born in the United States between 1990 and 1994. In the study, there were about 700,000 African-American women with children and the remainder, I believe, were Caucasian. When they looked at their birth weights, they found that even when they normalized the African-American women with the Caucasian women for educational standing, number of prenatal visits, and economic background, the children of the African-American women were smaller.

Another person did a study in which she took African-American children who did not have diabetes and compared them to Caucasian children without diabetes. During adolescence, all of us develop insulin resistance. The researcher checked these African-American children against Caucasian children during adolescence to see if African-American children had more insulin resistance, which predisposes us to Type 2 diabetes. And she found that was, indeed, true. Even before they had diabetes, African-American children had higher insulin levels, indicating that they might be insulin resistant. She did insulin-sensitivity studies and showed that African-American children tended to be more insulin resistant during adolescence compared to Caucasian children even before they developed diabetes.

If you put all of this together, the thrifty genotype, thrifty phenotype, and high insulin levels predispose these populations to diabetes. That is one of the reasons that the ADA came up with this recommendation in March 2000. Children belonging to these ethnic groups— Asian Indians, African-Americans, Hispanics, Pacific Islanders, Japanese-Americans—if they carry certain risk factors in terms of family history of diabetes at a young age or were above a certain percentile in height and weight, they would be considered high-risk. The recommendation is that from age ten every two years, that a child should have a fasting glucose test performed, because that child is at high risk for Type 2 diabetes.

Another problem being found now is that Type 1 diabetes children tend to be very thin. But because of obesity being so prevalent these days, we don't know if the children have Type 1 or Type 2 diabetes when they present to us. It's getting very complicated.

In your clinical practice, are you witnessing a greater incidence of diabetes in children?

I don't particularly see children, but occasionally I do. Someone asked me to see a boy about two or three weeks ago. The young boy came in with typical Type 1 diabetes symptoms. He was a very, very big kid. They asked me if he had Type 1 diabetes or Type 2. We checked him, for certain immune markers for Type 1 diabetes, and he was positive for those immune markers. That is what the ADA is recommending now, because in children, it is becoming a big problem to differentiate between Type 1 and Type 2. Pediatricians will tell you that they are seeing lots and lots of kids with diabetes, particularly among minorities.

The Role of Diet and Exercise

You talked about the genotypes. Does the expression of the genotype appear to be affiliated with prosperity and our economy?

I don't know if I would say prosperity per se. What I can say is diet. If you are prosperous or rich, you may actually have a better diet than if you are poor, where you are at times more at the mercy of fast-food chains.

That is a bigger problem. The food habits of our parents and ourselves, along with how much we exercise, influence our risk. Let's face it: many people who made huge profits on NASDAQ in 1999 and were able to retire would have all the time in the world to exercise every day and try to look good. Everybody else is working. If you have a desk job, you tend to eat a pizza and work through lunch, so how much exercise do you get?

I was born and raised in India, but I spent five years in Ireland and Europe. The first thing that struck me when I came to the United States is that people do not walk, because there is no place to walk. If you live in a housing development, what do you see? If you go to any housing development in Europe or India, they have these mom-and-pop shops, footpaths, and streetlights. In the evening, people walk to these places. In the United States, you don't have streetlights or footpaths. And commercial enterprise is not allowed in a residential area, so you have to get into your car and drive to the local supermarket. You get out of your car and go into the supermarket. If you want to get a movie to take home from the store nearby, you can't cross over because it is sealed off with barriers. You have to get into the car and drive over to the movie rental store.

All of this prevents exercise on a daily basis. If you talk to exercise experts, they will tell you that 30–45 minutes of exercise three times per week is enough for you. Often, we don't get even that.

And kids are often tied up with computer games after school.

Right. Parents are exhausted because they work. They often pick up pizza, and everybody in the family sits around and watches television. It is going to get even worse with Web television. All people will do is sit and vegetate.

Although we want to address the rising tide of diabetes among the

young, our readers often are confronted with adult-onset diabetes. If people
are concerned that they might have diabetes but know that it will take time
to keep an appointment with their physician, are over-the-counter, noninva-
sive testing kits useful in the initial diagnosis of diabetes?

They could be. We tend not to recommend urine testing at times because, from a scientific basis, there is a problem with what we call a tubular maximum, or T-Max, for glucose. There is a threshold in the kidneys before they start excreting glucose—that is, where you will be able to detect it. That T-Max tends to change with age. As you get older, your kidneys don't function as well, so the T-Max gets altered and your sugars might go very high before you actually start seeing it in the urine, which is a problem. But, yes, it is a way to do it. The over-the-counter finger-stick tests are very easy to do now, and many places now offer free glucose testing. The ADA has still not recommended universal screening. Maybe it will come to that. Right now, adults over the age of 40 should be screened for diabetes every three years. . . .

The Influence of Nature and Nurture

When we talk about the importance of lifestyle and diet on the emergence of
diabetes, it begs the question: Can diabetes be prevented through changes in
lifestyle?

The thought is that since genetics predisposes you to diabetes but does not actually cause diabetes—and since environment is a big factor in causing diabetes—clearly, if the environment can be modified, you may be able to prevent diabetes. The answer to this question will actually come out in the next two years. There is a big multicenter NIH-sponsored study that is ongoing called the Diabetes Prevention Program (DPP). This is exactly the question that they are trying to answer. Researchers have taken thousands of patients from across the country and have randomized them into protocols of putting them on a diet and exercise program, or giving them drugs before they have full-blown diabetes to see if one or more of these modifications can actually prevent diabetes from occurring. This is a question that everybody wants answered. They have put millions of dollars into this, and hopefully, we will have some answers in a few years.

You have mentioned specific genotypes in the predisposition to diabetes.
Will the completion of the map of the human genome help you in research-
ing the cause(s) of diabetes?

It is going to help, but being a polygenic disorder, it is going to be very difficult. There is not going to be a cure from a genetic basis for diabetes.

Is this a perfect example of the influence of nature and nurture in a
disease?

Absolutely. There is not going to be a cure, but maybe they will be able to identify risks. The problem is that there are so many genes, and the genes are different in different populations. Even within the non-Caucasian population, the genetic makeup is completely differ-ent. From the perspective of one's susceptibility to diabetes, each gene they have looked at is different, so it is a very, very complex area. Mapping will help in specific forms of diabetes that are related to single gene disorders, such as maturity-onset diabetes of the young. But those cases are very rare. The map will be helpful. It is a little complex, but we will have to wait and see.

Older people should then just be aware that if overweight, they should screen themselves for diabetes. Because the symptoms of diabetes could be associated with so many different disorders, is it hard to associate symp-toms, necessarily, with the possibility that you might have the disease?

Everybody needs to be screened beyond age 40 or 45 every three years. If you are in a high-risk population, start screening earlier.

THE "THRIFTY GENOTYPE" THEORY

Hilary King and Gojka Roglic

In the following selection, Hilary King and Gojka Roglic examine geneticist James V. Neel's "thrifty genotype" hypothesis. Neel hoped to explain why diabetes, a disease with genetic determinants and debilitating complications that should interfere with reproduction, continued to be so common. Neel's hypothesis suggests that a gene that allowed hunter-gatherers to store energy to be used in times of famine would lead to obesity, insulin resistance, and glucose intolerance in a modern society where the food supply was more regular. Some research of minority populations in developing countries tends to support his theory; when modernized, those with a limited genetic pool who once faced a harsh natural environment had a higher incidence of diabetes. Other research, however, has challenged Neel's theory, claiming that low birth weight, not genetic factors, contributes to the prevalence of diabetes. Although research has proven that many genes contribute to a predisposition to diabetes, Neel's theory continues to inspire further research into the causes of diabetes. King and Roglic are officers of the World Health Organization in the diabetes section of the Department of Noncommunicable Disease Surveillance.

"The problem of understanding the genetic nature of man is both a philosophical and, in these days of rapidly changing environment, a practical challenge. . . . In this essay an hypothesis has been advanced which envisions diabetes mellitus as an untoward aspect of a 'thriftiness' genotype which is less of an asset now than in the feast-and-famine days of hunting and gathering cultures."

It was in 1962 that the geneticist James V. Neel invoked a hypothesis to explain the apparent paradox that diabetes mellitus, thought to be genetically determined and environmentally triggered, should be common, despite sometimes presenting early in life and leading to severe consequences, which may interfere with reproduction—factors which should mitigate against its genetic selection. At that time dia-

From "Diabetes and the 'Thrifty Genotype,'" by Hilary King and Gojka Roglic, *Bulletin of the World Health Organization*, August 1999. Copyright © 1999 by *Bulletin of the World Health Organization*. Reprinted with permission.

betes epidemiology was in its infancy, but it was already known that the disease was particularly common among certain indigenous North American tribes. Neel proposed that a "thrifty" metabolism would confer a survival advantage to hunter-gatherer societies when faced with intermittent supplies of food, by permitting them to store excess energy in times of plenty, for subsequent utilization in times of want. In the modern setting, with regular food supplies, this thrifty metabolism would lead to a tendency towards obesity, insulin resistance and glucose intolerance.

Neel developed his proposal in the days before a clear distinction had been made between the pathogenesis of type 1 (also known as insulin-dependent) and type 2 (or non-insulin-dependent) diabetes. When, in due course, the hypothesis was applied selectively to type 2 diabetes, with its later onset and association with obesity and insulin resistance, it became more coherent and did much to stimulate early population studies of diabetes.

Studying Minority Populations

Diabetes epidemiology is unusual in that more information is available for developing countries, and the minority populations of the developing countries, than for most populations of European origin. A review of the available data has clearly demonstrated that type 2 diabetes occurs frequently (prevalence > 10%) among adults in a number of developing countries or among minority populations which fulfill the criteria for natural selection of thrifty genes—a formerly harsh natural environment and restricted ancestral genetic admixture, as well as their expression—recent socioeconomic modernization, with consequent impact on nutritional habits and exercise patterns. The result has been the development of obesity, insulin resistance and glucose intolerance, frequently with concomitant hypertension and hyperlipidaemia—a condition now most often referred to as the "metabolic syndrome." Latest projections predict a doubling of the number of people affected by diabetes over the next quarter of a century, from 150 million in the year 2000 to 300 million in the year 2025.

These findings have been broadly supportive of Neel's hypothesis, which has been reappraised on several occasions. One study even examined archaeological evidence and concluded that variation in susceptibility to diabetes among North American Indian tribes could be accounted for by the food preference (continued reliance on Arctic-style, unpredictable big game hunting, or generalized hunter-gathering) of the first wave of migrants (palaeo-Indians) after they moved southwards as the glaciers of the last ice age retreated. The authors concluded that the formative period for selection of the thrifty genes in these populations was approximately 11,000 years ago, when many big game species were becoming extinct in temperate North America. Indian groups which migrated eastwards or westwards along the ice margins did not have to adapt to a rapid and radical change of environment, and were not subject to such selection pressure.

As the epidemiological map of diabetes unfolds, it is becoming apparent that it is not the high prevalence, non-European populations which are unusual, but rather that European populations are unusual in their comparatively low prevalence of diabetes among adults. A symposium devoted to Neel's hypothesis, held in Auckland, New Zealand, in 1994, noted that it might be "Eurocentric" to treat European populations as the norm, and to look for explanations for the higher prevalence found in other ethnic groups. Rather, it might be useful to search for putative selection pressures which could account for a reduced susceptibility to type 2 diabetes in European populations. However, the review concluded that the thrifty genotype hypothesis remains helpful as an explanation of selection pressures which predispose to obesity, insulin resistance and glucose intolerance.

Challenging Neel's Hypothesis

Recently, fresh interest and attention has been brought to the subject by the work of C.N. Hales & D.J.P. Barker, who noted that low birth weight was associated with subsequent type 2 diabetes and cardiovascular disease in an English cohort. They proposed a "thrifty phenotype" hypothesis, which they consider a challenge to Neel's theory. It is also of note that adult Nauruans [a Polynesian people living on an island in the central Pacific Ocean], with their exceptionally high prevalence of type 2 diabetes, suffered great nutritional hardship during the Second World War, but subsequently became affluent. This could suggest a cohort effect of fetal and infant undernutrition, combined with an abundant food supply later in life, as a possible explanation for the recent epidemic of type 2 diabetes among Nauruans. Recently, a decline in the incidence of diabetes has been observed among Nauruans, which Hales & Barker attribute to improved fetal and infant nutrition among subjects born after 1945. However, the original investigators offered another explanation: a fall in the population frequency of the susceptible genotype due to the severity of the epidemic. A high prevalence of diabetes has also been observed among Ethiopian Jews who migrated to Israel after surviving famine conditions in their native country.

Among Pima Indians, who suffer from a prevalence of type 2 diabetes as high as that of Nauruans, both low and high birth weight have been shown to be associated with subsequent diabetes, although approximately 90% of Pimas with diabetes had a birth weight within the normal range. D.R. McCance et al. concluded that the association with low birth weight could be explained by the selective survival in infancy of low-birth-weight infants predisposed to insulin resistance, thus reinstating the genetic explanation.

Neel's hypothesis cannot be proven historically, and type 2 diabetes is now considered to be a polygenic disease, with different genes likely to confer susceptibility in different populations. However, as an ingenious explanation for a disorder which constitutes a major epidemic of our times, it has so far survived almost 40 years of critical appraisal. Thanks to its rival hypothesis, the debate has even intensified during the 1990s, during which it has increasingly centered around the underlying pathophysiological mechanism.

Whether for or against the thrifty genotype hypothesis, epidemiologists and other scientists are likely to continue to be inspired by it to study the frequency, etiology and pathophysiology of type 2 diabetes and associated disorders for some time to come. This ongoing research is probably Neel's greatest legacy.

THE RELATIONSHIP BETWEEN OBESITY AND DIABETES

Sarah Scott

Unhealthy eating habits and a sedentary lifestyle in North America have led to an epidemic of obesity, which contributes to the onset of type 2 diabetes, writes Sarah Scott in the following selection. Obesity, Scott explains, makes it difficult for the body to convert sugar into fuel; consequently, too much sugar builds up in the bloodstream, which can ultimately lead to type 2 diabetes. The causes of obesity are easy to identify, Scott observes. For example, too many people eat hamburgers and French fries and choose to drive rather than walk, or watch TV rather than enjoy outdoor activities. The rate of type 2 diabetes is growing among children, most of whom are obese as a result of these lifestyle choices. Although there is no cure for those diagnosed with diabetes, Scott reveals, a diet and exercise regimen can prevent the onset of the disease or delay the arrival of complications. Scott writes on women's medical issues for publications such as *Chatelaine*, a women's lifestyle magazine.

A week before her 37th birthday, Patricia R. was hanging out at home with her family in Woodbridge, Ontario, on her day off from her job as a grocery clerk. The phone rang. It was the doctor's office. She had gone for a thyroid test at her family's insistence as she had been feeling tired. The doctor's secretary laid it on the line: Patricia has high blood sugar and Type 2 diabetes—the kind linked to obesity. "I started crying," Patricia recalls. "Everyone says when you have diabetes, you end up dying." Her doctor's advice: lose weight—and a lot of it. Her mother said what mothers sometimes say in these situations: "I told you so." Patricia winces. "I am a big girl," she admits. "For years, my mother said, 'Watch what you eat. Try to lose weight.' She's right. If I had done those things, I wouldn't be in this situation today."

The Price of the Good Life

Mothers are often right. Patricia's disease, diabetes, is a ballooning epidemic caused largely by our unhealthy eating and living habits.

We have it easy: access to lots of high-calorie food—junky snacks and super-sized fast foods—plus a lifestyle that requires little or no physical exertion. "It's the good life," said Dr. Bernard Zinman, a diabetes specialist at Mount Sinai Hospital in Toronto. "But it's not so good." The result of this culture of overindulgence has become painfully obvious: a recent Health Canada survey found that 29 per cent of adults were obese (defined as having a body mass index of more than 27). That extra fat—especially abdominal fat—is a lot more dangerous than you might think. It can bring on Type 2 diabetes, the most common form of the disease. In fact, the survey found that 59 per cent of adult Canadians with diabetes were obese. Obesity hampers the body's ability to transform the sugar from food we eat into energy that fuels our cells. When that process malfunctions, too much sugar can build up in the bloodstream—identifying the chronic incurable condition called diabetes. Having high blood sugar is just the beginning: diabetics are vulnerable to a whole host of health complications, such as heart disease and kidney problems. And treating this epidemic and its secondary conditions costs the Canadian health-care system about $9 billion a year.

On a cold day in mid-February, Patricia is telling her story to 15 other men and women who have all been diagnosed with Type 2 diabetes, most within the past few months. "I'm very scared and very nervous," Patricia tells the group. They're gathered in this pale second-floor meeting room for a two-day course given by Tri-hospital Diabetes Education Centre (TRIDEC), Toronto's oldest diabetes education centre. They're going to learn how to mend their dietary ways and manage this lifelong condition. As they begin to tell their stories, you can hear the guilt, the denial, anger, anxiety and resigned jokes about the overindulgence that has contributed to their condition.

"I do most of the cooking," says Steven, a burly interior designer. "I cook for 12 and eat for 10."

"Are you married?" Patricia asks.

Steven laughs. He went to the doctor because he was tired all the time and literally falling asleep at his desk. "I used to be quite active. But on the weekends, I make a large breakfast and go back to bed for three hours."

Adam (a pseudonym), a muscular technician, regales the group with tales from Scotland, where he once lived. "Anything fried in the world you can find in Glasgow," he says fondly. Even Mars bars. Adam doesn't indulge in that kind of food anymore. He works out with weights, avoids salt, sugar and even alcohol. He walks everywhere. He was sure it was a mistake when the test showed his blood sugar was too high.

Beside Adam is a woman in a smart black pantsuit, white blouse and thin gold necklace. At 51, she has a busy job at a bank and sings in a choir. "I didn't have any symptoms," she says. She asked that her name be omitted because she doesn't want the bank to know about her diabetes: maybe it would be used as an excuse to hold off a promotion. But naturally, she told the ladies at lunch. "Four of us have diabetes. One is obese. One is overweight. Two are perfectly normal. But we're all in the same age bracket. The body starts to deteriorate."

"Don't say deteriorate," says Adam. "Say change."

"Well, in my case, it's deteriorate," she says, smiling weakly.

Eating Ourselves to Death

The causes of obesity are easy to identify and theoretically preventable, but they are frustratingly hard to address. Think of the pervasive North American lifestyle that offers up giant cups of soft drinks with the plateful of fries and the all-dressed quarter-pound hamburger at affordable prices. And then consider our sedentary life. We barely need to move anymore in a world where we take elevators instead of climbing stairs, drive to the store or school instead of walking, watch TV instead of playing in the park and sit at the computer firing off e-mails instead of getting up to do anything. It's believed that we burn about 800 fewer calories a day than adults did at the beginning of the 20th century, according to Dr. Julia Alleyne, medical director of SportC.A.R.E., a sports medicine department at Toronto's Sunnybrook & Women's College Health Sciences Centre.

This lack of everyday activity is a key contributor to the quick rise in Type 2 diabetes, experts believe. Inadequate exercise compromises the body's ability to use insulin effectively, which leads to an increase in blood sugar. "We're getting fatter; we're getting lazier. We do less," says Dr. Stewart Harris, a family physician and associate professor at the University of Western Ontario's Centre for Studies in Family Medicine in London. "The result is a growing epidemic of diabetes worldwide."

The type of food we're shovelling in may also partly explain the problem. After all, you don't get obese on broccoli. There's a controversial theory that blames our diet of highly refined carbohydrates, such as sweets and white bread, for the rise of diabetes. Because these carbs are quickly turned into sugar in the blood, the body is forced to churn out more insulin to absorb the extra sugar. Or so the theory goes. At some point, the body will not be able to keep up with the demand for insulin. Proponents of the theory, such as Dr. Thomas Wolever, a professor in the department of nutritional sciences at the University of Toronto, cite studies by the Harvard School of Public Health on the effect of diets with low fibre and a high glycemic index. The glycemic index (GI) ranks foods based on their immediate effect on blood sugar. Low-fibre high-GI diets increase the risk of developing Type 2 diabetes by as much as two to three times, the studies say. Yet, according to mainstream diabetes experts such as Dr. Zinman, the type of carbohydrates doesn't matter; obesity remains the problem.

Like Patricia, people who receive a sobering diagnosis of diabetes soon learn their condition won't ever go away. In fact, it will make them susceptible to a litany of health consequences that can be serious, even fatal—most notably cardiovascular disease. People with diabetes are two to four times more likely to suffer strokes or heart disease—one of the biggest killers of diabetics. And there's more to this depressing story. Diabetes is the leading cause of adult-onset blindness and end-stage renal disease. In addition, severe nerve damage can mean that diabetics may lose a limb to amputation.

A Growing Problem for Children

Experts estimate that more than two million Canadians have diabetes. The Centers for Disease Control and Prevention in the U.S. warned about "a major public health threat of epidemic proportions." In the 1990s, the number of diagnosed cases among American adults rose 33 per cent to hit 6.5 per cent of the adult population. No longer an old person's disease, it now affects people in their 40s, 30s and even in their 20s. Manitoba medical epidemiologist James Blanchard predicts that by 2015, 175,000 Canadians under age 40 will be afflicted. It's creeping into the world of children too, as increasing numbers of them get fat. This trend was first identified in North American native peoples, who have reported an alarming incidence of Type 2 diabetes in their kids. But now the problem has been reported in children from other ethnic groups at greater risk for the disease, especially kids who are obese or have a family member with diabetes. For example, a recent study of non-native Quebec youth found that 5 to 9 per cent had insulin resistance syndrome, a precursor to Type 2 diabetes.

The first Canadian case of a child with Type 2 diabetes was diagnosed in 1986, says Dr. Heather Dean, a pediatric endocrinologist in Winnipeg. It was a strange discovery; Type 2 diabetes was assumed to be an adult disease (indeed, we once called it adult-onset diabetes). The numbers grew quickly. Since 1986, about 200 kids in Manitoba and northwestern Ontario, the majority native people, have been diagnosed with Type 2 diabetes. Manitoba can now claim one of the largest groups of children with Type 2 diabetes in the world. "Eighty per cent of Type 2 diabetic kids worldwide are obese," Dr. Dean continues. "Almost all have at least one parent with diabetes." This troubling discovery shows that both genes and a dramatic change in lifestyle can pull the blood sugar trigger. After all, not all obese people develop diabetes, just those unlucky ones with a genetic predisposition. Some, particularly native people, have a genetic profile that makes them especially vulnerable if they eat a high-calorie diet and reduce their physical activity. And they have done so in many aboriginal communities in Canada and the U.S. over the past couple of generations. For example, the Oji-Cree of Sandy Lake, Ontario, were once a semi-nomadic people who hunted and trapped their own meat-heavy diet. Their metabolisms helped them weather periods of famine. Now, like other North Americans, they can feast every day and no longer need to exert themselves to survive. The frightening result: 26 per cent of the native people in Sandy Lake have diabetes, the third-highest recorded rate in the world.

From Here to Obesity

Patricia remembers when her weight started to balloon. Just after high school, she began working as a hairdresser in Toronto. She was a little overweight in high school—size 15 or so—but never obese. Then she started eating at fast-food restaurants. Cheeseburgers and fries were her favourites. She ate her way to a size 32—which probably helped her qualify for her job at a plus-size clothing store. Obesity doesn't run in the family; her sister, who owns a Mr. Sub franchise with fast food at her fingertips, has never had a weight problem; her mother is 20 pounds or so overweight. On top of her eating frenzy, Patricia didn't exercise either, at least not until she switched jobs last year and started working at a grocery store. With all the walking on the job, Patricia managed to lose 48 pounds by April and has gotten down a few sizes. But she's a little late.

"I walk all over the place," Patricia told her fellow diabetics in one of the sessions that TRIDEC holds as part of its two-day course. The lecturer, Dr. Alleyne, was impressed. Walking at a brisk pace for at least 30 minutes, she told the group, is a great way to get aerobic exercise. (Swimming, cycling and dancing are good too.) Exercise decreases the appetite and makes cells more sensitive to insulin, allowing glucose to be utilized more efficiently. It also reduces blood sugar and helps to lessen the severity of complications of diabetes. Patricia listened carefully. Her new exercise plan began a couple of days after the TRIDEC course ended, on the eve of her 37th birthday. "I kind of bent to the toes, up and down," Patricia says. She even got onto the cross-country ski machine for 10 minutes. Well, it's a start. But the next day, Patricia couldn't resist the party food; it was her birthday, after all. "We kind of pigged out," she says. "Baked potatoes, ribs, a piece of fruitcake with fresh peaches, kiwi and strawberries. Yeah, I cheated."

A diet-and-exercise regimen remains the cornerstone of treatment and control of Type 2 diabetes. But as any dieter knows, it's not easy to follow a restricted food plan, especially a permanent one. To control blood sugar, Patricia and the other diabetics learned at TRIDEC that they must eat a healthy diet that regulates the intake of carbohydrates from starch, fruit and vegetables and milk. Some diabetics can control their problem for a few years by eating well and exercising, delaying the need for drugs to control blood sugar. But even model patients will need drugs or insulin injections eventually, according to a major British study. "The problem with diabetes is that it's a silent disease," says Dr. Harris. "Nobody feels it. It doesn't hurt. That's why it's so hard to identify and so hard to treat."

A Pound of Prevention

If you can't get rid of diabetes, you do have a good shot at preventing it. To do so, we all need to take the same steps the TRIDEC gang will: eat healthily and incorporate exercise into our lives. But that's easier said than done in a culture of abundance where jumbo-size plates have become the norm. Realizing the need for prevention, the federal government has launched the five-year $5-million Canadian Diabetes Strategy to track the epidemic and promote a healthier lifestyle. Experts say we especially need to reach out to kids before they get big like the problem. But this is a challenge, especially when many schools are cutting physical education programs and tearing up playgrounds. In the U.S., where the percentage of young people who are overweight has almost doubled in the past 20 years, the Centers for Disease Control and Prevention offers this practical advice: walk your children to school. At snack and mealtime, make healthful foods widely available and discourage the consumption of those that are high in fat, sodium and added sugars. Heap praise on kids who make healthful eating choices, but "do not use food for reward or punishment of any behaviour."

If kids can start from scratch, adults need some remedial help in preventing diabetes. Dr. Harris says a key is to avoid gaining weight as your metabolism changes in your 30s, 40s and 50s. That means you have to make wise food choices and avoid excess fat and calories. But equally important, you should ensure you're incorporating daily activity into your life. So, walk to the store, Dr. Harris says. Walk your child to school. Climb the stairs instead of taking the elevator. "You don't have to join a health spa," says Dr. Harris. "I tell everyone with diabetes to go and get a dog."

STUDYING DIABETES IN THE PIMA INDIANS

Jane DeMouy

In 1963, researchers discovered a high rate of diabetes among the Pima Indians of southern Arizona. Since this discovery, writes Jane DeMouy of the National Institute of Diabetes and Digestive and Kidney Diseases (NIDDK), a branch of the National Institutes of Health, a cooperative effort between NIDDK researchers and Pima volunteers has led to significant discoveries about the causes and progression of diabetes and its complications. For example, DeMouy reports, researchers have learned that obesity and insulin resistance, strong predictors of diabetes, run in families; by studying the Pima Indians, researchers may find the genes that predispose some people to diabetes. As a result of the cooperation of the Pima Indians, the author observes, researchers and clinicians can identify those at risk for diabetes and its complications and begin preventive strategies such as improving diet and exercise and lowering blood pressure.

History paints a colorful portrait of the American Indians who live today in the Gila River Indian Community. Their ancestors were among the first people to set foot in the Americas 30,000 years ago. They have lived in the Sonoran Desert near the Gila River in what is now southern Arizona for at least 2,000 years.

Called the Pima Indians by exploring Spaniards who first encountered them in the 1600s, these early Americans called themselves "O'Odham," the River people, and those with whom they intermarried, "Tohono O'Odham," the Desert people.

Archaeological finds suggest that the Pima Indians descended from the Hohokam, "those who have gone," a prehistoric people who originated in Mexico. Strong runners, the Pima Indians were also master weavers and farmers who could make the desert bloom. Once trusted scouts for the U.S. Cavalry, the Pima Indians are pathfinders for health, helping scientists from the National Institute of Diabetes and Digestive and Kidney Diseases (NIDDK), a part of the National Insti-

From "Introduction," by Jane DeMouy, *The Pima Indians: Pathfinders for Health,* www.niddk.nih.gov, National Institute of Diabetes and Digestive and Kidney Diseases.

tutes of Health (NIH), learn the secrets of diabetes, obesity, and their complications.

Migrating from Mexico, the people settled the land up to where the Gila River and the Salt River meet, in what is now Arizona. They established a sophisticated system of irrigation that made the desert fruitful with wheat, beans, squash and cotton. The women of the community made exquisite baskets so intricately woven that they were watertight.

The Generosity of the Pima Indians

They were also a generous people. They sheltered the Pee Posh (or Maricopa Indians) who fled attack by hostile tribes, and who also became part of the Gila River community. Anyone who followed the Gila River, the main southern route to the Pacific, encountered these peaceful and productive traders who gave hospitality to travellers for hundreds of years. "Bread is to eat, not to sell. Take what you want," they told Kit Carson in 1846.

Today, the Pima Indians of the Gila River Indian Community are still an agricultural people, nurturing orchards of orange trees, pistachios and olives. They are still giving, too. Eleven thousand strong, the members of the Gila River Indian Reservation have participated in 30 years of research that will help people avoid diabetes, have healthier eyes, hearts, and kidneys, and to understand how and why people gain weight and what can be done to prevent it.

"The Pima Indians are giving a great gift to the world by continuing to volunteer for research studies. Their generosity contributes to better health for all people, and we are all in their debt," says Dr. Peter Bennett, Chief of the Phoenix Epidemiology and Clinical Research Branch of the NIDDK.

The Pima Indians' help is so important to the ability of doctors to understand and treat diabetes, obesity, and kidney disease because of the uniqueness of the community. There are few like it in the world.

Young Pima Indians often marry other Pimas. Many Pima families have lived in the Gila River Indian Community for generations. Because of this, scientists can search for root causes of disease through several generations of many families. The length of NIDDK's study and the number of families involved allows scientists an invaluable perspective on how the disease progresses. The more generations studied, the deeper and better the understanding of how diabetes affects people, and the greater the opportunity to develop drug or genetic therapy, or lifestyle changes that will slow or prevent the coming of disease.

The research takes so long, says NIH scientist Dr. Bill Knowler, because diseases like obesity and diabetes are so hard to understand. There seem to be several different causes, and the complex interaction between the genes a person inherits and the lifestyle a person chooses can make it hard to find treatments and cure. Scientists are trying to find a path through this maze.

Thirty years of research show that exercising and eating lower fat, fiber-rich foods can at least delay diabetes. "If you delay it long enough," adds Dr. Knowler, "it's almost as good as preventing it."

This cooperative search between the Pima Indians and the NIH began in 1963 when the NIDDK (then called the National Institute of Arthritis, Diabetes and Digestive and Kidney Diseases), made a survey of rheumatoid arthritis among the Pimas and the Blackfeet of Montana. They discovered an extremely high rate of diabetes among the Pima Indians. Two years later, the Institute, the Indian Health Service, and the Pima community set out to find some answers to this mystery. They hoped to shed light on an even broader question: Why do Native Americans, Hispanics and other non-white peoples have up to ten times the rate of diabetes as Caucasians?

A Productive Effort

Three decades' collective efforts by scientists and volunteers have laid the foundation for eventually curing or preventing diabetes and its complications. The work begun in 1965 has yielded a definition of diabetes that is now used worldwide, and set out diagnostic criteria used by doctors from Sacaton, Arizona, to Sicily to identify and treat diabetes and to anticipate how it is likely to develop.

Doctors can best treat a disease when they understand what causes it and how it progresses. By studying Pima volunteers for many years, NIH doctors learned that unhealthy weight is a strong predictor of diabetes. Eighty percent of people with diabetes are overweight. They also discovered that high levels of insulin in the blood, or hyperinsulinemia, is another strong risk factor.

Studying this clue, researchers working with patients found that high levels of insulin were linked to insulin resistance. Normally, the pancreas releases insulin to regulate the amount of sugar or glucose in the blood. People who have non-insulin-dependent or Type II diabetes (hereafter referred to simply as "diabetes") produce insulin, but their bodies don't respond to it effectively. NIH researchers have made it clear that people with insulin resistance are those most likely to get diabetes.

By studying Pima Indian volunteers, Dr. Clifton Bogardus and his colleagues established that glucose not needed for immediate energy is converted to glycogen and stored in skeletal muscle. However, several enzymes that drive this natural process appear different in insulin resistant people, according to the researchers, and they continue to study the biochemistry of insulin resistance to understand this breakdown and how it might be repaired.

Looking for Genetic Clues

By studying Pima Indian volunteers, researchers have determined that diabetes runs in families, as does insulin resistance, and obesity. Scientists believe that some people also have a gene that makes them more likely to have the kidney disease that occurs in people who have had diabetes a long time. Looking for these genes is a key part of the search now being conducted by NIH and the Pima Indians.

Researchers are working on this complex genetic puzzle by studying blood drawn from every member of the Pima community who comes into the NIH clinic at Hu Hu Kam Memorial Hospital for an examination. Blood is checked for healthy levels of blood sugar, cholesterol and other nutrients. Then, each person's blood and serum are typed and some is reduced to a very small pellet of DNA, the genetic material that instructs a person's cells to function one way or another. When NIH researchers find a family with one parent who is diabetic and one who is not, they are able to study the genes of both parents and their children in an effort to find the gene or genes shared by those who have diabetes.

After finding these genes, scientists hope to break the codes that cause insulin resistance, obesity, diabetes and kidney disease of diabetes. "If we can locate the genes contributing to disease—some enzyme being made or not being made," explains Dr. Knowler, "we can identify which people are at high risk for the disease and figure out ways to intervene." Finding these genes will help doctors identify youngsters at risk and begin prevention before disease sets in.

Another important finding has already made a difference in how diabetes patients are treated. The complications that come with long-term diabetes—kidney disease, eye disease, and amputations caused by nerve damage—are the major reasons for illness and death among the Pima Indians. When Dr. Knowler began his research in Phoenix, few understood what he and his colleagues would discover by working with Pima volunteers: that high blood pressure predicts complications of diabetes such as eye and kidney disease, and that lowering blood pressure may slow the onset of diabetes and the progress of already existing kidney disease. Because of this work, doctors today are not only aware of the need to treat high blood pressure in people with diabetes, but they begin treating it sooner than in the past.

"Our greatest pride," says Dr. Knowler, "is in conducting research that affects clinical practice."

Looking Forward

Other research with important implications for future generations is Dr. David Pettitt's study of high blood sugar and diabetes in pregnant women. By working with Pima volunteers, Dr. Pettitt found that children born to diabetic women are more likely to be overweight and more likely to develop diabetes than children of women who have not developed diabetes.

Dr. Eric Ravussin conducts studies that measure food intake, metabolism, and energy expenditure to evaluate their interaction and contribution to a genetic predisposition to obesity.

Now NIH and the Pima Indians are building on these accomplishments. "The search goes forward on two fronts," says Dr. Knowler. "We're working hard on the genetics of the disease. We're optimistic we will find one or more genes. It's still hard to predict how we might prevent diabetes, but we might, for example, be able eventually to correct the genetic difference that causes disease. More immediately, identifying the diabetes genes would allow us to identify the people most likely to get the disease."

The second strategy is to encourage those who are at high risk to change behaviors that can lead to diabetes, such as eating a high fat diet, being physically inactive, and being overweight.

The NIH has begun a major nationwide program to prevent diabetes in people who increase exercise and eat lower fat foods. Fifty percent of the volunteers will be American Indians and other minorities, and once again, the Pima Indians will be prominent among them. Health for this and future generations: that's the NIH-Pima goal.

DIABETES AND AGENT ORANGE: A CONTROVERSIAL LINK

Gina Kolata

A U.S. Air Force report released in March 2000 links exposure to high levels of dioxin, the main chemical in Agent Orange, to the incidence of diabetes, reports Gina Kolata in the following selection. Air Force statisticians conducted a study of Vietnam veterans, comparing those who participated in the spraying of the defoliant Agent Orange to those who did not. The increased incidence of diabetes was discovered when comparing the levels of dioxin. According to the author, critics of the study note that dioxin is stored in fat; the study fails to distinguish whether the diabetes was caused by high dioxin levels or obesity, a factor known to contribute to diabetes. Despite criticism of the study, Kolata notes, the government will likely compensate victims who develop diabetes. Kolata is a science reporter for the *New York Times*.

An Air Force report raising questions about whether the defoliant Agent Orange might be linked to diabetes in Vietnam veterans is as puzzling as it is provocative.

The study [released in March 2000] compared the health of 859 veterans of Operation Ranch Hand, in which the defoliant Agent Orange was sprayed on much of the landscape during the Vietnam War, to that of 1,232 who did not spray the chemical. There was no difference in the incidence of diabetes in the two groups—16.9 percent of the Ranch Hand group was diabetic and 17 percent of the control group was diabetic.

The diabetes effect only showed up when scientists looked at the levels of dioxin, the main chemical in Agent Orange, in the men's blood. After adjusting for factors like age and body fat levels, they concluded that the Ranch Hand participants with the lowest levels of dioxin in their blood had a 47 percent lower risk of diabetes than those with the highest levels of dioxin in their blood.

Veterans not involved in Operation Ranch Hand showed the same trend, said Dr. Joel E. Michalek, an Air Force statistician who is the

From "Agent Orange and Diabetes: Diving into Murky Depths," by Gina Kolata, *New York Times*, March 30, 2000. Copyright © 2000 by The New York Times Company. Reprinted with permission.

principal investigator for the study. Most people have some dioxin in their blood because it was once widely used as a herbicide, so people were exposed to it in the environment, and it persists in body fat.

Dr. Michalek said in a telephone interview that the two groups of Air Force veterans might have shown no difference in their diabetes incidence, over all, because many men in the Ranch Hand group did not have high dioxin levels. About half of the Ranch Hand group, he said, had average levels of the defoliant in their blood. So even if dioxin exposure did increase diabetes risk, the effect might not have been apparent. For that reason, he said, his group moved on to advanced statistical modeling and data analyses.

He added, though, that other scientists had questioned the Air Force findings and methods.

A Questionable Link

A major criticism of the Air Force study, Dr. Michalek said, has been that it is hard to sort out a dioxin effect from an effect of simply being overweight.

Dioxin is stored in fat, so the fatter a person is, the higher his dioxin levels are likely to be. But the fatter someone is, the more likely he is to develop diabetes. The question scientists asked was, is the effect due to dioxin or to obesity?

"We know diabetes is highly related to body fat, and so is dioxin," Dr. Michalek said. "That's why these diabetes findings are so difficult to interpret. People are concerned that we haven't done the right body fat adjustment."

Dr. Michalek said he and his colleagues first started seeing a link between Agent Orange and diabetes in 1991. Though "the findings were met with criticism in the scientific community," he said, Air Force researchers have continued to see the effect, even after searching assiduously for other factors that might have explained it away.

He said that the Air Force considered the March 2000 report's statistical analysis the strongest evidence yet, but that it was beginning two additional biochemical studies to see if the effect held up. He added that the service had asked the federal government to spend millions of dollars on more such studies.

Dr. Michalek said that no matter how he adjusted for other factors, like age, body weight and family history of diabetes, the association between dioxin exposure and diabetes remained. But some scientists are skeptical.

Among them is Dr. Michael Gough, a retired biologist who was chairman of a federal advisory panel for the Ranch Hand study from 1990 to 1995. After spending years on the dioxin question, Dr. Gough said, "The conclusion I've come to is that there is no evidence whatsoever to support any connection between low-level dioxin exposure and any human disease."

Some statisticians said the Air Force study was fraught with pitfalls. Among them is the fact that Vietnam veterans have linked a variety of health complaints to exposure to Agent Orange and the study aims to look at virtually all of them.

"This study is unprecedented," Dr. Michalek said. "We have so many end points."

But, as statisticians point out, that makes it very likely that something will turn up by chance alone, making it especially difficult to sort out whether an effect is real.

Dr. David Freedman, a statistician at the University of California, says he grows wary when a study looks at large numbers of possible outcomes and then makes complicated statistical adjustments to come up with a positive finding for one of them. "The more types of funny analyses you see, the more your antennae can be quivering," he said.

At this point, Dr. Michalek said, he is unwilling to say whether he thinks that dioxin really does cause diabetes. "I am a scientist," he said, explaining that he is awaiting results from the biochemical studies.

Looking for Compensation

Some veterans, however, say it is time that the Department of Veterans Affairs compensates them if they develop diabetes.

"Based on the evidence we have seen, the V.A. [Veterans Administration] should make a decision that diabetes is presumed to be service-connected based on Agent Orange exposure," said John Sommer, executive director of the Washington office of the American Legion.

Dr. Gough, for one, said he did not doubt that the veterans would end up being compensated for diabetes.

"I think there is a feeling in this country that the Vietnam veterans got a bad shake, and I don't deny for a minute that that was true," Dr. Gough said. "That has now extended to the constant suggestion that Agent Orange poisoned the men."

Despite the questions about the Air Force study that plague many scientists, Dr. Gough said, "I'm certain that diabetes will be turned into a compensable disease for Vietnam veterans."

CHAPTER 3

THE PREVENTION
AND TREATMENT
OF DIABETES

Contemporary Issues
Companion

PREVENTING AND TREATING TYPE 2 DIABETES: AN OVERVIEW

Anita Smith

Although the number of people diagnosed with type 2 diabetes has risen to epidemic proportions, the disease is both preventable and treatable, writes Anita Smith in the following selection. The author reveals, for example, that women who develop gestational diabetes can alter their diet to prevent complications. In addition, maintaining a low fat diet combined with exercise can minimize the risk of developing diabetes later in life. According to the author, a program of diet and exercise is an important tool in preventing the onset of type 2 diabetes, particularly for the growing number of children who are developing the disease. Furthermore, researchers continue to develop better drugs to lower insulin resistance, improved tests to measure glucose levels, and innovative tools to make monitoring glucose less painful.

The future is brighter every day for people with diabetes. Researchers are learning more about this disease and developing innovative treatments that make it easier to manage. Yet more Americans than ever— a diverse group of 16 million—have diabetes. And the number continues to grow.

A Preventable Epidemic

Diabetes has risen at a startling rate: 30 percent in the 1990s. More than 90 percent of people who have diabetes are classified as type 2, which until the late 1990s mostly occurred in overweight adults older than 45. Today, however, the disease does not discriminate. Women and men in all races and ethnic groups, along with children and adolescents, are developing type 2 diabetes.

The epidemic of type 2 diabetes seems linked to a major risk factor: obesity, or being overweight by about 30 or more pounds. The rate of obesity in the United States has increased by 57 percent since 1991. Simply put, Americans sit too much and eat too many fatty foods. They pay a heavy price: spiraling health-care costs and, for those with diabetes, a lifetime of potential complications, including blindness, kidney failure, heart attack, and stroke.

The statistics seem grim. But they are reversible. Type 2 diabetes is preventable, and certainly treatable, especially when you exercise and stick to a low-fat diet.

Some diabetes risk factors, such as heredity, cannot be controlled, says David S.H. Bell, M.D., of the University of Alabama at Birmingham. These factors include having a close relative with diabetes, such as a father, mother, sister, or brother; or being of African-American, Latino, Native American, or Asian descent. Or, you might have high blood pressure, "good" (HDL) cholesterol that is too low (less than 40 mg/dl), or triglycerides (another type of fat in the blood) that are high (more than 259 mg/dl).

A Special Concern for Women

About 8.1 million women and about 7.5 million men have diabetes. There's a higher incidence of type 2 diabetes in women than in men probably because females tend to be more overweight, says Bell.

Women are vulnerable to other risk factors, such as having given birth to a large baby. "By that, I mean a baby weighing more than 10 pounds," says Bell.

Some women develop gestational diabetes, which occurs in 2 to 5 percent of all pregnancies. However, it disappears when a pregnancy is over. A registered dietitian, working with the doctor, can plan a diet that provides the baby with adequate nutrition while omitting foods that increase blood sugar levels in the mother. Women with gestational diabetes may avoid insulin injections if they do not eat certain foods, such as table sugar, honey, brown sugar, corn syrup, maple syrup, molasses, soft drinks, fruit drinks, fruit packed in syrup, cake, cookies, ice cream, candy, jams, and doughnuts. It is also recommended that fruit juices be limited to 6 ounces and taken with meals.

About one-third of women with gestational diabetes will develop type 2 later on, says Bell. Many of these women can prevent this from happening if they keep their weight down—after pregnancy—by following a diet low in fat and calories, and exercising.

If you are a diabetic woman who wants to bear children, seek expert medical advice before getting pregnant. "Generally, it's better for pregnancy to occur when you're younger and in the early, controlled stages of diabetes," says Bell. "However, you'll need high-risk pregnancy management, which might include an endocrinologist working with your obstetrician."

Women with diabetes, especially type 2, are at risk for heart problems. "Women who are not diabetic typically do not get heart disease until they're in their 60s," says Bell. "However, with diabetic women, this can occur a lot earlier." That's why it's essential that their doctors apply what Bell calls the Big Three: (1) Treat the blood sugar problems associated with diabetes; (2) treat lipids—the cholesterol and triglycerides; and (3) keep blood pressure under control.

A Crisis for Children

Traditionally, pediatricians have treated type 1 diabetes in children, not type 2. Type 1 diabetes has been called "juvenile diabetes" and type 2 "adult-onset diabetes." But those lines are blurring because of an increase of type 2 diabetes in children and adolescents. This crisis is an indictment of our lifestyle—too much junk food and television and too little exercise, says James R. Gavin III, M.D., of the Howard Hughes Medical Institute in Chevy Chase, Maryland, and a former president of the American Diabetes Association.

Parents can fight this epidemic by exercising with their children and minimizing fast-food junkets. Stock the fridge with fruits and vegetables, and put beans, grains, cereals, low-fat dairy foods, lean meats, chicken, and fish on the family menu.

If your children have diabetes, ensure they get cholesterol and other blood fat tests, a yearly dilated eye exam, a foot exam to check circulation and nerves, a urine test to check kidney function, and regular dental checkups. They need to have their blood pressure checked regularly; if elevated, it should be treated.

Using Better Tools

"There now are tremendous drugs to treat type 2 diabetes," says Bell. "We've got drugs, such as Actos (pioglitazone) and Avandia (rosiglitazone), that lower insulin resistance, and drugs, such as Starlix (nateglinide) and Prandin (repaglinide), that help the pancreas make more insulin."

The hemoglobin A1c test, a valuable but underused tool, makes a big difference in treatment. The test can tell the doctor how high the patient's blood sugar has been on average over the last two to three months. This provides a better picture of the degree to which the kidneys, heart, nerves, and eyes have been exposed to high blood sugar.

Surprisingly, only 40 percent of patients with diabetes get the hemoglobin A1c test once a year, says Bell. If you are diabetic, talk to your doctor about taking the test.

Developing Painless Possibilities

For those who must take insulin, the chore of injection has gotten quicker and less painful with inventive gadgets. For example, a disposable, penlike injector that contains insulin and small needles tucks in a pocket.

The insulin pump, an improved insulin-delivery method used mainly by type 1 diabetic patients, is available in sizes as small as a pager.

All patients with diabetes must measure blood glucose with finger-stick tests—on a daily basis or even hour by hour—so they know how food, exercise, and medication affect their blood sugar. But the days of numerous pricks and sore fingers may end soon, thanks to new testers. The Food and Drug Administration has approved a meter resembling a wristwatch that uses low-frequency electrical current to measure glucose. Other products under development include a patch that continuously monitors glucose levels, and a self-monitoring device with a laser to draw blood.

The insulin inhaler is another innovation. However, more studies are needed to investigate how inhaling insulin directly into the lungs affects lung tissue, says Bell. Gavin does not believe these inhalers will replace insulin injections for most patients over the long term.

For now, medications, regular checkups, nutrition, and exercise are the best ways to manage diabetes, and live a full life.

THE PREVENTION AND TREATMENT OF CHILDHOOD DIABETES

Allen M. Spiegel

Children who suffer from diabetes must endure lifelong treatment, says Allen M. Spiegel, director of the National Institute of Diabetes and Digestive and Kidney Diseases (NIDDK). In the following excerpt from congressional testimony delivered on June 26, 2001, at a hearing on childhood diabetes, Spiegel reviews the research objectives established by the NIDDK, a branch of the National Institutes of Health (NIH) whose goals include alleviating the burden faced by diabetic children and their families. For example, Spiegel states that one objective of research is to uncover the genetic determinants of diabetes and the environmental factors that trigger the disease in those who are genetically predisposed to it. Once the risks are identified, Spiegel reports, continuing research into pancreatic islet transplantation, replacing damaged insulin-producing beta cells, offers hope of a cure that will alleviate the burden of daily insulin injection and expensive pancreas transplants. Since very young children have difficulty recognizing the symptoms of low blood sugar, says Spiegel, the resulting seizures and loss of consciousness can be very frightening; therefore, the institute also supports the development of glucose management technology to improve the quality of life for diabetic children and their families.

One of the most important health care issues facing our Nation is the increasing burden of diabetes. According to the Centers for Disease Control and Prevention (CDC), diabetes affects an estimated 16 million Americans, including both genders, the young and the old, all races and ethnic groups, the rich and the poor. Consistent with the topic of today's hearing, I will focus my testimony on diabetes in children, who, in many ways, suffer most from the disease. They have the disease from an early age and must endure lifelong treatment. They must carefully adjust what they eat and everything they do—from

Excerpted from Allen M. Spiegel's congressional testimony before the Senate Permanent Subcommittee on Investigations, Government Affairs Committee, during the 2001 Children's Congress, June 26, 2001.

schoolwork to sports—in order to manage their disease. Even with a continuous struggle to follow such regimens, they may still develop serious, long-term complications of diabetes.

A Widespread Problem for Children

Approximately one million Americans have type 1 diabetes, which is typically diagnosed in childhood, adolescence or young adulthood. They must have daily insulin administration to survive, and must monitor their blood glucose levels throughout the day and night. While the value of maintaining blood glucose control in preventing or delaying the onset of complications has been demonstrated through National Institutes of Health (NIH) research, this therapy is extremely difficult and is not without risks.

We are also very concerned about reports that more and more children are being diagnosed with type 2 diabetes. While patients with type 2 diabetes usually do not lose all of their insulin-producing ability and thus may not require insulin administration, they are susceptible to the same complications as those with type 1 diabetes.

The NIH has established a broad consultative process to frame a productive diabetes research agenda for fiscal year (FY) 2001 and beyond. . . . We are focusing our research agenda for type 1 diabetes around six important goals: to understand the genetics and epidemiology so that we can identify who is at risk for developing diabetes, to prevent or reverse the disease, to develop cell replacement therapy as a true cure for diabetes, to prevent or reduce hypoglycemia (low blood sugar) which limits tight control of blood sugar, to prevent or reduce complications, and to attract new research talent to the field.

Understanding the Genetics of Type 1 Diabetes

Type 1 diabetes has strong genetic determinants; over the last few years, several genes have been linked to type 1 diabetes, and several chromosomal regions have been identified that harbor additional genes that confer susceptibility to type 1 diabetes. The National Institute of Diabetes and Digestive and Kidney Diseases (NIDDK) is launching major new research initiatives related to the genetics of type 1 diabetes, in conjunction with the National Institute of Allergy and Infectious Diseases (NIAID), the CDC, and the Juvenile Diabetes Research Foundation International (JDRF). We are forming an International Type 1 Diabetes Genetics Consortium to analyze genetic data from U.S., European and Australian family collections. These data have the potential to identify the additional genes that confer susceptibility for type 1 diabetes. A related research initiative will expand efforts to establish a central repository of genetic data relevant to type 1 diabetes and provide an Internet-based information service for researchers through the International Histocompatibility Working Group.

We are also stepping up research to uncover the environmental "triggers" that, in combination with a genetic predisposition, may make some individuals especially prone to developing the disease. In order to understand the interplay of genetic and environmental factors in type 1 diabetes more fully, the NIDDK is bolstering research on the epidemiology of the disease, in collaboration with the CDC, the NIAID, the National Institute of Child Health and Human Development (NICHD), and the National Institute of Environmental Health Sciences (NIEHS). One project will establish a large population of siblings, children and parents of individuals with type 1 diabetes to identify genetic and environmental causes of the disease. By studying the interaction of genes, the environment and the immune system, we may be able to identify factors that trigger the onset of autoimmunity in type 1 diabetes—the destructive process in which the body's immune defense system destroys its own insulin-producing cells. Given that type 1 diabetes may have its roots very early in life, another project will identify newborns genetically at risk for type 1 diabetes and follow them through the high-risk age (from 0 to 15 years) to identify additional genetic and environmental causes. Research will be expanded at several sites, including Colorado, Florida and Washington. The CDC and NIDDK are also supporting a population-based registry to define the prevalence and incidence of diabetes in children. This project, entitled "SEARCH," will identify all children with diabetes in six regions of the country and will help us understand trends in disease development.

Genetic clues can also be derived from animal models, which are an essential tool for understanding health and disease in humans. They help clarify the function of genes and provide systems for testing possible treatments that are not yet ready for human trials. Widely used animal models of diabetes include the non-obese diabetic (NOD) mouse and the BB [Bio Breeding] rat.

The foregoing genetic and epidemiologic studies should facilitate identification of those at high risk for development of type 1 diabetes. This in turn will allow us to intervene in an effort to prevent the disease. To spur the testing of promising new strategies to prevent or delay progression of type 1 diabetes, the NIDDK, in collaboration with the NIAID and NICHD, is creating a clinical trials network, the "Type 1 Diabetes TrialNet," a major recommendation of the Diabetes Research Working Group. To develop a therapeutic or preventive vaccine, the NIH is actively pursuing research along several fronts. The NIDDK supports basic research to facilitate the establishment of a solid knowledge base enabling the selection, development and testing of promising candidate agents for the treatment and/or prevention of type 1 diabetes. Building on this knowledge base, the NIAID and NIDDK will be launching a program with the long-range objective of developing prevention strategies, including vaccines for autoimmune diseases, with emphasis on type 1 diabetes. This new research program is being co-sponsored by NICHD, the National Institute of Dental and Craniofacial Research (NIDCR), the National Institute of Arthritis and Musculoskeletal and Skin Diseases (NIAMS), the NIH Office of Research on Women's Health (ORWH), and the JDRF.

Developing Cell Replacement Therapy

Cell-based therapy offers the hope of a real cure for type 1 diabetes and would be far superior to the two current alternatives: daily insulin administration or whole pancreas transplantation. Insulin administration via multiple daily injections or through an insulin pump is an extraordinarily difficult therapy and a poor substitute for the body's own finely tuned mechanism for releasing insulin only at the times and in the amounts necessary to maintain normal blood glucose levels. Whole pancreas transplantation is also problematic. It is major surgery, is usually done only in conjunction with a kidney transplant, and is not a feasible therapy for young children. In contrast to these current treatments, cell-based therapy would have many advantages for patients, including ease of administration—an important factor in the medical treatment of children.

Gaining knowledge about the genes of the insulin-producing beta cells of the pancreatic islets is also critical to combating type 1 diabetes. These cells are the key to insulin production and resulting glucose control. Thus, a new initiative will support the development of a gene expression array—a tool used to analyze which genes are turned "off and on" under different conditions, including diabetes. We expect that this research will provide important insights about possible new molecular targets for the treatment and prevention of type 1 diabetes.

Advances have sparked an exciting wave of new hope that a cure for type 1 diabetes can be realized through pancreatic islet transplantation. The crest of that wave is a promising study in Edmonton, Alberta, Canada, in which islet transplantation permitted a small number of people with type 1 diabetes to remain healthy for over a year without daily insulin injections. The NIH is now expanding clinical studies to exploit and extend these impressive findings. One major NIH effort, the Immune Tolerance Network (ITN), is a consortium of research institutions, led by the NIAID, which seeks to replicate the successful results of the Edmonton protocol in a larger number of patients.

In complementary research, the NIDDK, in conjunction with the Department of the Navy, has established a Transplantation and Autoimmunity Branch, in which several islet transplants have been performed in adult patients with severe type 1 diabetes. The Walter Reed Army Medical Center and the University of Miami's Diabetes Research Institute are also collaborating in this research. The National Center for Research Resources (NCRR) also plans to establish up to six islet isolation centers across the U.S. to coordinate procurement of pancreatic tissue, isolation of islets, and their distribution for use in research protocols. These centers would also perform research and development to improve islet isolation techniques. In addition, the NIDDK will support an islet/beta cell transplant registry to collect data from all institutions performing islet and beta cell transplants in North America. As islet transplantation continues to be perfected, we will need to address two issues that could limit its widespread clinical application: (1) inadequate supplies of islets and (2) imperfect methods to prevent transplant rejection. We have several initiatives under way to resolve these issues.

Addressing the Limits of Islet Transplants

First, we are accelerating research on many aspects of beta cell development and function so that we can increase supplies of donor pancreatic tissue for transplantation, possibly by developing alternative sources of islet beta cells. With NIDDK leadership, the NIH is taking a significant step in the development of cell-based therapy by establishing a comprehensive beta cell project, as recommended by the Diabetes Research Working Group. The consortium approach will provide scientists with access to information, resources, technologies, expertise, and reagents that are beyond the means of any single research effort. A comprehensive understanding of the molecular basis of beta cell development and function will then help to generate new research tools and to provide critical insights into the prevention and treatment of type 1 diabetes. Another approach to cell-based therapy is research on laboratory-generated replacement cells.

Second, we are supporting research on alternatives to the lifelong immunosuppressive drug treatments that are currently required to prevent rejection of transplanted islets and kidneys. One innovative research program, led by the NIAID and NIDDK, is developing methods to induce immune tolerance to transplanted kidneys and islets in non-human primates so that the grafts will be accepted by the recipient's immune system without the need for global immunosuppression. Because of the similarities between the human and non-human primate immune systems, results from this program will directly influence studies in the Immune Tolerance Network, TrialNet, and other NIH and JDRF supported clinical trials in islet and kidney transplantation. Such novel approaches to educating the immune system not only increase the likelihood of achieving a true cure for type 1 diabetes, but may also offer hope of preventing the disease in those at risk. Through these combined efforts, we are hopeful that islet transplantation can become the real cure we are all seeking for patients with type 1 diabetes, many of whom are children and young adults.

Preventing or Reducing the Complications of Type 1 Diabetes

The medical management of children with type 1 diabetes is particularly challenging. The occurrence of low blood sugar is a major factor limiting the ability to achieve good metabolic control and thus reduce the risk of complications. Very young children cannot be taught the symptoms of low blood sugar or to alert their parents to take action when sugar levels drop dangerously low. Symptoms of severe low blood sugar can include seizures or loss of consciousness, which can be very frightening and may cause permanent problems. The NIDDK, in conjunction with the National Institute of Neurological Disorders and Stroke (NINDS), the National Institute of Nursing Research (NINR), NICHD and the JDRF, is expanding research to understand the pathways involved in being aware of hypoglycemia, and clinical research on methods to reduce or prevent hypoglycemia.

The complications of diabetes affect virtually every system of the body. Diabetes is the leading cause of kidney failure, new blindness in adults, and non-traumatic amputations. It is a major risk factor for heart disease, stroke, and birth defects; shortens average life expectancy by up to 15 years; and costs the nation in excess of $100 billion annually in health-related expenditures. The NIDDK, in collaboration with the National Eye Institute (NEI), NIDCR, NHLBI, and NINDS, is supporting numerous initiatives to reduce and prevent the complications of diabetes. We are increasing research efforts to identify new targets for therapy. We are encouraging the development of surrogate markers for clinical trials by expanding the study of how genes function in tissues commonly involved in diabetes complications and by the development of improved diagnostic techniques. The NEI is initiating clinical trials relevant to diabetic eye disease. Several promising new drugs are under development to prevent diabetic eye disease and other complications involving the small blood vessels. We are also working to identify genes that may increase susceptibility for the development of the eye and kidney complications of diabetes.

Attracting New Talent to Research

In order to accelerate the pace of research, a cadre of exceptionally talented and dedicated researchers is needed to bring the power of their intellects and expertise to bear on understanding, treating, preventing and curing type 1 diabetes. As the base of fundamental knowledge about type 1 diabetes grows, the opportunities also increase to translate this information into new diagnostic, preventive and therapeutic strategies. The NIDDK is supporting initiatives to foster the development of "bench to bedside" research through a partnership of both basic and clinical scientists in order to bring discoveries in the laboratory more rapidly to a clinical setting in which the patient can benefit. In addition, we are encouraging diabetes researchers to act as "talent scouts" to identify leading scientists with expertise or cutting-edge technology and bring them into type 1 diabetes research. New awards will support partnerships between such scientists and type 1 researchers.

I am grateful for the opportunity to share with you these examples of the many exciting NIH research efforts directed toward conquering diabetes in children. Diabetes places a tremendous burden on patients and their families, especially when it strikes in childhood. Through research, we will find the means of lifting the strain of this disease from their shoulders. Today, there is an unprecedented sense of enthusiasm and momentum in the diabetes community. We are eager to pursue the many scientific opportunities made possible by the biotechnology revolution. We are encouraged by the dedicated efforts of patients and their families, by organizations such as the Juvenile Diabetes Research Foundation International, and by the Diabetes Caucus.

DIET, EXERCISE, AND DRUG TREATMENT DELAY TYPE 2 DIABETES

Joan Chamberlain and Jane DeMouy

In the following selection, Joan Chamberlain and Jane DeMouy of the National Institute of Diabetes and Digestive and Kidney Diseases (NIDDK) discuss the Diabetes Prevention Program (DPP), a national clinical trial that compared the effectiveness of diet and exercise to drug treatment in delaying the onset of diabetes in people who have impaired glucose tolerance, a condition which often precedes the disease. The authors describe the study's participants, explain its methods, and summarize its conclusions. According to the authors, although the drug metformin reduces the risk of diabetes, "lifestyle intervention" including a low-fat diet and exercise can reduce the risk of getting type 2 diabetes by 58 percent. While researchers do not know how long lifestyle changes will delay the onset of diabetes, they believe that the results represent a major step toward containing diabetes, which has become a national epidemic.

At least 10 million Americans at high risk for type 2 diabetes can sharply lower their chances of getting the disease with diet and exercise, according to the findings of a major clinical trial announced by U.S. Department of Health and Human Services (HHS) Secretary Tommy G. Thompson on August 8, 2001, at the National Institutes of Health (NIH).

"In view of the rapidly rising rates of obesity and diabetes in America, this good news couldn't come at a better time," said Secretary Thompson. "So many of our health problems can be avoided through diet, exercise and making sure we take care of ourselves. By promoting healthy lifestyles, we can improve the quality of life for all Americans, and reduce health care costs dramatically."

The same study found that treatment with the oral diabetes drug metformin (Glucophage®) also reduces diabetes risk, though less dramatically, in people at high risk for type 2 diabetes.

Participants randomly assigned to intensive lifestyle intervention

From "Diet and Exercise Dramatically Delay Type 2 Diabetes: Diabetes Medication Metformin also Effective," by Joan Chamberlain and Jane DeMouy, National Institute of Diabetes and Digestive and Kidney Diseases, August 6, 2001.

reduced their risk of getting type 2 diabetes by 58 percent. On average, this group maintained their physical activity at 30 minutes per day, usually with walking or other moderate intensity exercise, and lost 5–7 percent of their body weight. Participants randomized to treatment with metformin reduced their risk of getting type 2 diabetes by 31 percent.

The Diabetes Prevention Program

The findings came from the Diabetes Prevention Program (DPP), a major clinical trial comparing diet and exercise to treatment with metformin in 3,234 people with impaired glucose tolerance, a condition that often precedes diabetes. On the advice of the DPP's external data monitoring board, the trial ended a year early because the data had clearly answered the main research questions.

Smaller studies in China and Finland have shown that diet and exercise can delay type 2 diabetes in at-risk people, but the DPP, conducted at 27 centers nationwide, is the first major trial to show that diet and exercise can effectively delay diabetes in a diverse American population of overweight people with impaired glucose tolerance (IGT). IGT is a condition in which blood glucose levels are higher than normal but not yet diabetic.

Of the 3,234 participants enrolled in the DPP, 45 percent are from minority groups that suffer disproportionately from type 2 diabetes: African Americans, Hispanic Americans, Asian Americans and Pacific Islanders, and American Indians. The trial also recruited other groups known to be at higher risk for type 2 diabetes, including individuals age 60 and older, women with a history of gestational diabetes, and people with a first-degree relative [parents, brothers, sisters, and children] with type 2 diabetes.

"Lifestyle intervention worked as well in men and women and in all the ethnic groups. It also worked well in people age 60 and older, who have a nearly 20 percent prevalence of diabetes, reducing the development of diabetes by 71 percent. Metformin was also effective in men and women and in all the ethnic groups, but was relatively ineffective in the older volunteers and in those who were less overweight," said DPP study chair Dr. David Nathan of Massachusetts General Hospital, Boston.

DPP volunteers were randomly assigned to one of the following groups:

- intensive lifestyle changes with the aim of reducing weight by 7 percent through a low-fat diet and exercising for 150 minutes a week.
- treatment with the drug metformin (850 mg twice a day), approved in 1995 to treat type 2 diabetes.
- a standard group taking placebo pills in place of metformin. The latter two groups also received information on diet and exercise.

A fourth arm of the study, treatment with the drug troglitazone combined with standard diet and exercise recommendations, was discontinued in June 1998 due to the potential for liver toxicity.

DPP participants ranged from age 25 to 85, with an average age of 51. Upon entry to the study, all had impaired glucose tolerance as measured by an oral glucose tolerance test, and all were overweight, with an average body mass index (BMI) of 34. About 29 percent of the DPP standard group developed diabetes during the average follow-up period of 3 years. In contrast, 14 percent of the diet and exercise arm and 22 percent of the metformin arm developed diabetes. Volunteers in the diet and exercise arm achieved the study goal, on average a 7 percent—or 15-pound—weight loss, in the first year and generally sustained a 5 percent total loss for the study's duration. Participants in the lifestyle intervention arm received training in diet, exercise (most chose walking), and behavior modification skills.

Can the interventions prevent diabetes altogether? "We simply don't know how long, beyond the 3-year period studied, diabetes can be delayed," says Dr. Nathan. "We hope to follow the DPP population to learn how long the interventions are effective." The researchers will analyze the data to determine whether the interventions reduced cardiovascular disease and atherosclerosis [narrowing and hardening of the arteries], major causes of death in people with type 2 diabetes.

"Every year a person can live free of diabetes means an added year of life free of the pain, disability, and medical costs incurred by this disease," said Dr. Allen Spiegel, director of the National Institute of Diabetes and Digestive and Kidney Diseases (NIDDK), which sponsored the DPP. "The DPP findings represent a major step toward the goal of containing and ultimately reversing the epidemic of type 2 diabetes in this country."

Diabetes afflicts more than 16 million people in the United States. It is the main cause of kidney failure, limb amputations, and new onset blindness in adults and a major cause of heart disease and stroke. Type 2 diabetes accounts for up to 95 percent of all diabetes cases. Most common in adults over age 40, type 2 diabetes affects 8 percent of the U.S. population age 20 and older. It is strongly associated with obesity (more than 80 percent of people with type 2 diabetes are overweight), inactivity, family history of diabetes, and racial or ethnic background. Compared to whites, black adults have a 60 percent higher rate of type 2 diabetes and Hispanic adults have a 90 percent higher rate.

The prevalence of type 2 diabetes has tripled in the last 30 years, and much of the increase is due to the dramatic upsurge in obesity. People with a BMI of 30 or greater have a five-fold greater risk of diabetes than people with a normal BMI of 25 or less.

Managing Blood Glucose Combats the Complications of Diabetes

Shai Gozani

Diabetics suffer from numerous long-term complications that can result in blindness, heart attack, stroke, kidney failure, and the amputation of toes and feet. In the following selection, Shai Gozani discusses the nature of these complications and explains why managing blood glucose levels can reduce or slow their progression. The author stresses the importance of glucose monitoring and explores new technology that may alleviate the painful and frequent finger pricks that often prevent diabetics from monitoring their glucose. Efforts at understanding diabetes, says Gozani, may lead to better treatment and, perhaps, a cure. Gozani is a research fellow and instructor at the Harvard-M.I.T. Division of Health Sciences and Technology.

To J.M., a peaceful and uninterrupted night's sleep is something to cherish. All too often, this 54-year-old woman has her sleep shattered in the middle of the night by a painful burning sensation in her legs. In addition to these distressing incidents, J.M. can no longer feel her toes; they have been overtaken by a blunt and unyielding numbness.

What rare nervous system disorder afflicts J.M.? Actually, she suffers from one of the most common diseases in the United States: J.M. is one of an estimated 14 million Americans with diabetes mellitus, often referred to simply as diabetes. The abnormal sensations she experiences are characteristic of a relatively common complication called diabetic neuropathy.

What is diabetes and how does it affect the nervous system? Can it be treated and what does the future hold? These are questions that diabetics, as well as scientists, physicians and biomedical engineers, ask themselves daily.

Diabetes occurs in two predominant forms: Insulin-dependent diabetes mellitus (IDDM, type I) accounts for about 5 to 15 percent of cases and tends to arise in children and teenagers. However, the vast majority of individuals with diabetes—about 12 million—have non-insulin-dependent diabetes mellitus (NIDDM, type II) which often develops in the fourth or fifth decades of life.

The cardinal feature of diabetes is an abnormal metabolism of the blood sugar known as glucose. Insulin, a hormone normally produced by the pancreas, is largely responsible for the regulation of glucose levels in the blood. Diabetics either lack insulin or have a resistance to the action of the hormone. This absolute or relative insulin deficiency prevents them from properly metabolizing glucose and leaves them with chronically high concentrations of glucose in their blood, or "hyperglycemic." Most evidence indicates that the long-term health consequences of diabetes are caused by persistent hyperglycemia.

Damaging the Nervous System

Long-term complications of diabetes are numerous. One of the most characteristic is called retinopathy, or disease of the retina. In fact, diabetic retinopathy is the leading cause of blindness in the United States. Another, nephropathy, or kidney disease, occurs in a significant number of diabetics; about 25 percent of individuals with kidney failure requiring dialysis and/or kidney transplantation have diabetic nephropathy. Diabetics also suffer from a greater than normal rate of heart attacks and stroke.

Many individuals who have had either type of diabetes for more than five to 10 years will suffer from diabetic neuropathy. Those who experience symptoms of diabetic neuropathy often consider these the most distressing manifestations of their diabetes.

The most common expression of diabetic neuropathy is a loss of sensation in the feet and occasionally in the hands. Beyond the disturbing and troublesome numbness, a lack of sensory feedback from the feet can trigger a sequence of dangerous events. In particular, the malfunction of nerves carrying sensory information from the feet may lead to an altered foot architecture that increases the probability of injuries of which the individual is unaware. These injuries may develop into foot ulcers, or craterlike lesions of the skin that are often infected. In some cases, the ulcers do not heal and amputation of damaged toes, or even the entire foot, is required—a devastating situation striking all too many individuals who have had diabetes for many years.

For reasons that are not well understood, a minority of diabetics experience knifelike or burning sensations in their extremities in addition to, or in place of, the loss of sensation in diabetic neuropathy. At times, these painful sensations are severe enough to cause a further complication, clinical depression.

Another common target of diabetic neuropathy is the autonomic nervous system where it can produce highly disruptive alterations in basic functions, including the digestive, bladder and sexual functions.

In fact, impotence eventually affects more then 50 percent of men with diabetes.

Managing Blood Glucose Levels

While there is no cure for any form of diabetes and few effective treatments for its specific complications, a fairly effective treatment paradigm is emerging. The Diabetes Control and Complications Trial (DCCT) validated what many endocrinologists have believed for years. It demonstrated that very aggressive attempts to normalize blood glucose levels reduce the likelihood or rate of progression of several long-term complications of diabetes.

For nerve disease, the study showed that participants whose blood glucose levels were intensively managed had a greater than 50 percent reduction in all manifestations of diabetic neuropathy after five years. Although the DCCT was limited to individuals with insulin-dependent diabetes, the results are believed extensible to non-insulin-dependent diabetes.

It is important to say that normalization of blood glucose levels in diabetics has risks. Intensive blood glucose management such as that utilized in the DCCT tends to increase the probability of severe hypoglycemia, characterized by rapid drops of the blood glucose concentration. Hypoglycemic events are dangerous and may result in coma if not rapidly reversed. As a result, intensive blood glucose management requires increased medical supervision and attention by the diabetic.

The whole purpose of managing and improving blood glucose levels is to lower the chronically high amounts of glucose that diabetics tend to have in their blood. This reduction in glucose concentration is accomplished through regulation of diet, exercise, weight loss if appropriate, and the administration of therapeutic agents such as insulin. To insure treatment efficacy and safety, especially with intensive management, frequent determinations of blood glucose levels are required. As a result, "self blood glucose monitoring" by diabetics has become a fundamental component of diabetes management. Diabetics who attempt to aggressively normalize their blood glucose require three or more glucose checks a day.

Improving the Technology

Since 1986, technologies that facilitate blood glucose monitoring have advanced significantly. Diabetics can carry a small device, not much larger than a credit card, that allows them to check their glucose level by placing a drop of blood on a special test strip inserted into the "glucose meter." The blood droplet is usually obtained by pricking one's finger tip with a small lancet. This technology has revolutionized blood glucose monitoring, but for patients whose diabetes might most demand it, multiple "finger pricks" extract a significant toll.

Many diabetics consider the finger prick painful and highly onerous, and compliance with the recommended monitoring frequency is quite low. In fact, many individuals refuse to use the monitors at all. Children and the elderly have a particularly difficult time with the compliance and use of the current technology. As a result, tremendous efforts have been directed at creating a "noninvasive" and painless blood glucose monitor. Unfortunately, the development landscape for such a device has been repeatedly littered with the dashed hopes of diabetics. No such instrument is presently approved for public use.

Yet, there is cause for optimism. Several different noninvasive blood glucose monitoring technologies are under investigation, and there is good reason to believe that within five years the FDA will approve a truly effective and safe device. In addition, other approaches to treating the disease have made gains. Improvements in pancreatic organ transplants have led to their increasing role in the treatment of diabetes; recent advances in the design of an artificial pancreas have been encouraging, as have been improvements in automated insulin-delivery systems.

Beyond these developments, great strides are being made in understanding the fundamental causes of the various forms of diabetes and attendant complications, including diabetic neuropathy. Insights gained from this research may lead to new treatments and, possibly in the future, a cure. Hopefully, this knowledge will help J.M. sleep a little more peacefully.

TREATING TYPE 2 DIABETES IN WOMEN

Harvard Women's Health Watch

Women are more likely than men to develop diabetes, write the editors of *Harvard Women's Health Watch*, and as a result are at greater risk for one of the disease's complications: heart disease. In the following selection, the authors discuss the nature of diabetes and the factors that appear to make diabetic women more likely to have cardiovascular disease, such as high blood pressure and obesity. Experts suggest diabetic women be treated with cholesterol-lowering drugs. According to the authors, diet and exercise have also been known to reduce the complications of diabetes. For example, the authors report, losing ten pounds can return blood sugar levels to normal, and exercising five times a week can reduce the risk of developing diabetes. *Harvard Women's Health Watch* is a publication of current women's health reports by doctors of the Harvard Medical School.

If you're over age 40 and overweight, and you don't get enough exercise, you are at risk for type 2 diabetes, the most common form of this disease. That has particularly ominous implications for women, because they not only are more likely to develop the disease than men are, they also are disproportionately affected by its complications. Women with diabetes are seven times more likely to die of heart disease than nondiabetic women. For diabetic men, the equivalent increase in risk—while serious enough—is only two- to three-fold. Diabetic women also have a significantly higher incidence of congestive heart failure compared with diabetic men. When it comes to heart disease risk, diabetes completely erases a woman's premenopausal advantage over men.

Researchers do not yet know all the mechanisms involved in type 2 diabetes. It is far more complicated than was once thought, involving many genes, organs, and metabolic functions. Fortunately, treatment options have grown along with our recognition of its complexity. The best news in recent years is how effective diet and exercise are in preventing diabetes and reducing its severity.

The Basics of Diabetes

Diabetes develops when glucose can't get into cells and instead builds up in the bloodstream. Our bodies need glucose—a simple form of sugar that supplies energy to the cells—in order to function properly. The main source of glucose is food, mostly carbohydrates that break down to sugar in the intestine and cause blood glucose levels to rise. In response, the pancreas releases the hormone insulin, which directs glucose from the blood into the cells, either for immediate use or to be stored in fat and muscle. In so doing, insulin returns blood glucose levels to normal.

Type 1 diabetes, an autoimmune disorder that destroys the insulin-producing capacity of the pancreas, usually develops in childhood or adolescence. In type 1, the body cannot produce enough insulin to drive glucose into the cells, causing blood glucose levels to rise. Type 2 diabetes most commonly starts in adulthood. In this form of the disease, the pancreas makes plenty of insulin, but fat, muscle, and other cells resist the normal action of insulin—a condition called insulin resistance. This leads to elevated blood glucose levels (hyperglycemia). As part of the same process, the liver produces additional sugar, as well as triglyceride-rich lipoproteins, which raise LDL (bad) cholesterol and lower HDL (good) cholesterol. Blood pressure rises, and abdominal fat increases. These changes occur in both sexes, but particularly so in women.

Ninety percent of all diabetics have type 2 diabetes. Genetics, aging, and some medications can cause insulin resistance, but the main non-genetic factors are overweight and lack of exercise. Of the 800,000 Americans who will be diagnosed with type 2 diabetes this year, 90% will be overweight. How excess weight causes insulin resistance is unknown, but recent research suggests that fat cells secrete a hormone dubbed resistin that interferes with insulin action.

Insulin resistance alone is generally not enough to lead to clinical diabetes because the pancreas can compensate for a long time by pumping out more insulin. But eventually the pancreas becomes exhausted and cannot continue to produce high levels of insulin. As a result, glucose builds up in the blood and causes problems throughout the body. In the short term, diabetes can cause fatigue, nausea, frequent urination, increased thirst, and blurred vision. Uncontrolled, diabetes damages both large and small blood vessels, resulting in cardiovascular disease, blindness, kidney failure, and nerve disease.

Women, Diabetes, and Heart Disease

Women with diabetes tend to have cardiovascular risk factors that are more pronounced. For instance, the Strong Heart Study of cardiovascular disease in American Indians found that women with diabetes had greater increases in blood pressure and upper body obesity, higher levels of LDL cholesterol, and lower levels of HDL cholesterol than their male counterparts. Some researchers suspect that high blood glucose interferes with the heart-protective effects of estrogen. But how insulin resistance actually causes these malfunctions is not known.

According to new guidelines issued in May 2001 by the National Cholesterol Education Program (NCEP), women with diabetes are at as great a risk for heart attack as women who already have heart disease. Experts advise aggressively treating high cholesterol in such women with cholesterol-lowering drugs such as statins.

Treating Type 2 Diabetes

Weight loss—by way of exercise, diet, or both—is essential in treating type 2 diabetes. Losing 10 pounds can mean a return to normal blood sugar levels, even if you are significantly overweight. Weight loss lowers insulin resistance and helps your body use its insulin more efficiently.

For people with diabetes, staying active lowers the risk for cardiovascular disease, contributes to weight reduction, and helps use up glucose, which lowers blood glucose levels. And it increases insulin sensitivity, the opposite of insulin resistance. Exercise may also be the best way to prevent diabetes. The Harvard-based Nurses' Health Study and Physicians' Health Study have found, respectively, that women and men who exercise at least 5 times per week are about 40% less likely to develop diabetes than those who don't exercise.

Dietary control of diabetes centers on eating healthy meals and snacks on a regular schedule and shunning excess calories. Several studies have shown that fiber also helps. In 2001, research in the *New England Journal of Medicine* found that a high-fiber diet (50 grams per day) lowered blood sugar levels by 10%. That compares favorably with the effects of some currently available drugs.

While diet and exercise are the cornerstones of type 2 diabetes prevention and treatment, people with diabetes sometimes need medication as well.

Until fairly recently, the only oral diabetes drugs in the United States were sulfonylureas, medications that drive down blood sugar levels by increasing insulin production. When they failed, insulin injections were required. The years 1996 to 2001 have seen a big change. The number of medications has more than tripled and whole new classes of drugs have been introduced. In 2001, diabetes drugs address insulin resistance and production as well as high blood sugar levels. Doctors not only have a wider range of drugs to choose from, they also use them more aggressively.

If medications are inadequate, insulin injection is still the most effective therapy. Several companies are developing an inhaled form of insulin.

Traditionally, clinicians have used one treatment at a time for type 2 diabetes. If one therapy failed, another was substituted or added. But this approach succeeded in controlling blood sugar levels for only about a quarter of all patients. Now physicians are treating diabetes more effectively with multiple drugs in combination. This generally means lower doses of each individual drug and fewer side effects.

The most commonly used oral drug combination is metformin and a sulfonylurea, but other combinations are being tested. In 2000, researchers at Tulane University reported that a combination of metformin and rosiglitazone was better than metformin alone in improving blood sugar control, insulin sensitivity, and pancreatic cell function. Even if insulin shots become necessary, use of an oral drug as well can mean lower insulin doses.

Some diabetes experts also recommend that medications be started immediately—in conjunction with diet and exercise—rather than waiting to see if lifestyle changes alone will control blood sugar levels.

HEALTH PROFESSIONALS MUST PROMOTE NEW DIABETES TREATMENT OPTIONS

Christopher D. Saudek

Although diabetes can be treated, to do so diabetics must actively think about their disease twenty to thirty times a day, writes Christopher D. Saudek, president of the American Diabetes Association and director of the diabetes center at the Johns Hopkins School of Medicine in Baltimore. For this reason, Saudek argues, any medications or technologies that can improve the life of diabetics should not be dismissed because they appear too complicated or too expensive. Health-care professionals must support these advances because they have great potential to reduce the toll the disease takes on the people who must struggle with its complications.

Sometimes, inside the health-care professions and health-care regulatory agencies, we hear the opinion that type 2 diabetes isn't that big a deal. It isn't cancer and it isn't AIDS. It's just a lifestyle disease. People shouldn't have let themselves get overweight. There are lots of pills available, and then there's always insulin. It is amazing how often physicians don't even bother to tell people that they have diabetes; they soften the message with euphemisms like, "We'll have to watch your sugar," or the oldest of all, "You only have a touch of diabetes."

A Costly, Devastating Disease

Statistics do not support this casual attitude. Available through the American Diabetes Association's Web site, www.diabetes.org, the numbers are sobering: 15.7 million people have diabetes in the United States, and about 5.4 million don't even know it. Over 200,000 people will die of diabetes this year [2002]. About 15 percent of diagnosed people already have long-term complications when they are first told they have diabetes, and the mean time between onset and diagnosis is estimated to be seven years. Type 2 diabetes is the leading cause of end-stage renal disease, preventable amputations, working-age blind-

From "A 'Touch' of Diabetes?" by Christopher D. Saudek, *FDA Consumer*, January/ February 2002.

ness, and a major cause of heart disease and stroke. It cost over $98 billion in the United States in 1997. The stats go on, and paint an ugly picture of inadequate treatment with devastating results.

But isn't diabetes easily treated? Isn't it a disease people can easily take care of, if they would only pay attention? "Easily" is a huge misconception. It may be easy to say, "Diet and exercise, give up on the sweets, check your numbers, know your blood pressure and cholesterol and stop smoking, have your eyes checked, your feet, your lipids and your A1c [a test that measures average blood sugar levels over the previous three months]. Oh yes, and keep losing the weight." But have you, the reader, ever tried to take such good care of your health? Probably only if you have diabetes.

Adding things up, people with diabetes are expected to think about their disease perhaps 20 to 30 times a day, between worrying every time they eat, exercise, check their blood sugar or take a medication.

Supporting New Ways to Treat Diabetes

As new medications and new technologies are developed, it is worth thinking about what they mean for the person with diabetes. The new is too often dismissed by a summary comment: "Too expensive;" "a convenience item;" "too complicated for the average patient;" "not proven to be better." These put-downs were probably used when disposable syringes replaced boiling glass syringes, when ultrafine needles replaced thick needles. (I talked with a person the other day who had found the pan her deceased mother used to boil her glass syringe.) Better drugs, better meters, insulin pens and pumps translate into better self-care and fewer complications. And "too complicated" almost never applies: very little is too complicated for the average patient, and they need all the help they can get.

What about too complicated for the health-care professional? Those of us specializing in diabetes may be able to keep the medication options and the monitoring guidelines reasonably straight in our minds. But when diabetes is only a small part of a person's professional practice, it does present a huge challenge. In my opinion, the best thing to come along in the treatment of diabetes is the Certified Diabetes Educator, or CDE. It is a whole profession of people trained and certified in helping people with diabetes take care of themselves. People with diabetes and physicians who care for them should take advantage of the CDE.

So if diabetes is so complicated, so difficult to manage for the patient and health-care professional alike, is there any point trying? The evidence all points to a resounding "Yes." Large, definitive clinical trials such as the Diabetes Control and Complications Trial and the United Kingdom Prospective Diabetes Study have proven conclusively that not only do blood glucose control and control of other risk factors matter, but they are achievable.

I believe, therefore, that it is up to us in the health-care professions and the health segment of the government to keep pushing the medications and the technologies forward. A safe, reliable pill to help people lose weight, regardless of whether it independently affects blood glucose, would have an enormous effect in controlling diabetes, since obesity-related insulin resistance is the major underlying cause of type 2 diabetes. Thousands of people with diabetes will benefit from any new medication that some people will respond well to, that has fewer side effects, or that will keep some people off insulin for a while longer. Dramatic advances like continuous or non-invasive blood glucose monitoring will come gradually and incrementally.

It must always be remembered that the cost of diabetes is in the complications and in the personal toll it takes. The incremental expense of new drugs and new technologies makes up a relatively small part of the total cost of diabetes. We therefore have to continue the progress in making safe, effective drugs and devices available until treatment is as easy as taking an aspirin a day.

THE ADVANTAGES AND DISADVANTAGES OF USING INSULIN PUMPS

Robert S. Dinsmoor

Not unlike the pancreas, insulin pumps deliver small amounts of insulin to the body steadily over time. After the Diabetes Control and Complications Trial revealed that intensive insulin therapy could substantially reduce the risk of several major complications of diabetes, sales of pumps mushroomed. In the following selection, Robert S. Dinsmoor describes contemporary insulin pumps and explores their advantages and disadvantages. For example, he writes, evidence shows that those who use insulin pumps have less fluctuation in blood glucose, which minimizes the dizziness and other problems associated with abnormally low blood glucose. On the other hand, says Dinsmoor, because a part of the device must actually enter the body, the entry site can sometimes become infected. For most, however, the lifestyle flexibility the pumps provide outweigh any disadvantages: Pump users can eat and exercise more like nondiabetic people without losing control of their blood sugar levels. According to the author, however, only those who understand the nature of their disease and how certain foods and activities influence blood glucose levels should use pumps. Robert S. Dinsmoor is a writer from Massachusetts and longtime contributor to *Countdown* magazine, a publication of the Juvenile Diabetes Research Foundation.

Insulin pumps have come a long way since they were first introduced more than 20 years ago, and their popularity is soaring. The number of pump users in the United States climbed from 20,000 in 1995 to 80,000 in 1999. What's the appeal? For many people with Type 1 diabetes, insulin pumps add flexibility to lifestyle and help improve blood sugar control. While insulin pumps may not be the right choice for everyone with Type 1 diabetes, they are certainly becoming a viable option for more and more patients.

The Pump Comes of Age

When Colby Smith, 29, of Juneau, Alaska, recently considered pump therapy, he was haunted by unpleasant memories of previous pumps he'd had—like the Auto-Syringe he started lugging around back in 1979, when he was just a kid. It was cumbersome, and so heavy it broke his belt, so he had to start wearing it in a backpack. And it was temperamental—just having a little water splashed on it caused it to malfunction.

Other early pump users had their own complaints: Motors that spontaneously shifted into overdrive, delivering dangerous amounts of insulin; a lack of sophisticated programs or adequate alarms to warn users of problems; crude, uncomfortable infusion sets; or tubing that got blocked and stopped delivering insulin—or cracked and leaked insulin—the problem often not becoming apparent until blood sugars skyrocketed.

The idea behind the device was sound—to deliver insulin in a way that is physiologically similar to the way a nondiabetic pancreas does. Pumps infuse small amounts of insulin steadily over time (the basal infusion), just like the pancreas. Pump users can also deliver a bolus of insulin—that extra shot of insulin similar to what the pancreas secretes in response to meals. But clearly, the earliest models needed work.

Fortunately, throughout the 1980s manufacturers gradually made the pumps smaller, easier to use, technically more sophisticated, and safer. Yet, despite all the improvements, interest in the pumps had waned by the early 1990s, and most of the manufacturers had dropped out of the competition, leaving only two insulin pump manufacturers in the United States—MiniMed Technologies and Disetronic Medical Systems.

Perceptions about insulin pump therapy began to change after the results of the landmark Diabetes Control and Complications Trial (DCCT) were released in 1993. The study showed conclusively that intensive insulin therapy, using either insulin pumps or multiple daily insulin injections, could greatly reduce the risk of diabetes-related nerve disease, retinal disease, and kidney disease. (On the downside, those on intensive insulin therapy had three times as many episodes of severe hypoglycemia—low blood sugar levels—as those on conventional insulin treatment.)

Since the results of the DCCT were released, sales of insulin pumps have increased dramatically. The number of pump users in the United States mushroomed from about 11,400 in 1992 to roughly 80,000 in 1999. Further, those who start on pumps now tend to stay on them. The dropout rate—the percentage of pump users who eventually discontinue pump therapy—has declined from an estimated range of about 6 to 18 percent in the mid-1990s to a rate of about 2 to 3 percent in 2000.

In fact, the market for pumps is so strong, a new insulin pump manufacturer entered the competition. In February 2000, Animas

Corporation received approval from the Food and Drug Administration (FDA) to market its pump, the Animas R-1000 Insulin Pump, in the United States.

In their present incarnation, insulin pumps are only about the size of a beeper or a deck of cards, and weigh only 3.5 to 4 ounces. Each pump includes an infusion set with a thin plastic tube 24 to 42 inches long, one end of which is connected to an insulin reservoir in the pump and the other to a thin needle or plastic catheter (also called a cannula). The cannula is injected under the skin in the abdomen using an "inserter needle," which operates in much the same way as a standard syringe. However, when the inserter needle is removed, the cannula remains in position—inserted beneath the skin. An adhesive patch helps to secure the infusion set and cannula. The infusion set is usually removed and replaced in a new position every two to three days. Infusion sets have improved greatly in terms of comfort, and some now come with quick-release mechanisms for such activities as bathing, swimming, exercising, and sex.

Contemporary insulin pumps are also easier to use than earlier versions. Pump users can program many different basal rates throughout the day, and some pumps have "square wave" boluses—boluses that are spread out over time to match the timing of prolonged meals.

The Pumper's Advantage

Although conclusive evidence is lacking, many diabetes experts believe insulin pumps offer better blood sugar control than multiple daily injections (MDI). Whereas an MDI regimen supplies insulin in relatively large doses throughout the day, pumps continuously deliver insulin in small amounts—just like the pancreas does—resulting in less fluctuation in blood glucose. Moreover, the intermediate and long-acting insulins used in MDI regimens are absorbed somewhat unpredictably into the bloodstream, whereas the regular insulin infused by insulin pumps is absorbed much more predictably.

Yet, perhaps the most important and clear-cut advantage of pumps is flexibility: Most MDI regimens require patients to inject insulin and eat at pre-set times each day to correspond to the action profiles of the insulins used, whereas pumps deliver stable amounts of insulin, and patients can choose when to receive their mealtime boluses.

"Patients on pumps can be much more flexible in the timing of things," explains Ruth Farkas-Hirsch, R.N., C.D.E., a diabetes clinical specialist from the Diabetes Care Center at the University of Washington in Seattle. "They can sleep late, eat at different times, spontaneously engage in physical activity, or go to a party and graze all evening. They're able to enjoy daily life much more like a nondiabetic person, without losing control of their blood sugar levels."

Like those on MDI, however, people using insulin pumps must monitor their blood glucose levels at least four times a day—before each meal and at bedtime. This information is an essential component of tight blood sugar control, and helps pump users fine-tune their insulin delivery.

Very active people tend to benefit most from the flexibility of pump therapy. Before starting on his pump a year ago, Kevin Dombroski, 18, of Ansonia, Connecticut, had to eat right before his basketball, soccer, and golf games to avoid hypoglycemia. Now, he unhooks the pump for his basketball and soccer games and turns down his basal rate when he plays golf. "I thought it was going to be more complicated, but it actually makes my life a lot easier," Dombroski says.

The Down Side of Pumps

The most common complication of pump therapy, which occurs in about 30 percent of users, is infection at the site where the cannula pierces the skin. Users can minimize this risk by changing the syringe and tubing every two days or so and keeping the skin around the area clean.

Another potential risk is a disruption in the flow of insulin, leading to hyperglycemia (high blood sugar levels) and possibly even a life-threatening condition called ketoacidosis. This disruption can occur due to the pump malfunctioning, the tubing becoming kinked, or the tubing or catheter becoming blocked. It can be especially worrisome if it occurs at night, while the user is asleep. Insulin pumps now feature alarm systems to alert patients of possible blockages, reducing much of the risk associated with disrupted insulin flow.

For some people, the pump's biggest drawback is that it must be constantly "hooked up" to the body. Still, pumps are smaller and more portable than ever before, and they can be worn on one's belt, in one's pocket, or under one's clothes. In the age of ubiquitous beepers and cell phones, insulin pumps don't tend to get noticed as much. Nonetheless, for some, the thought of being "plugged into a machine" 24 hours a day can be oppressive.

Jeanne Going, 41, of Tucson, Arizona, decided to give pump therapy a try in the early 1990s and says she found it to be a "real nuisance." It was difficult to wear with clothes; when she got out of bed it fell and had to be reprogrammed; her abdomen was "just getting eaten up" by the tape; and her blood glucose control was excellent with or without it. She discontinued pump therapy about a year later (to the benefit of a young friend with Type 1 diabetes who "inherited" Going's insulin pump).

For other patients, the benefits clearly outweigh the disadvantages. "I was nervous about wearing the pump all the time, thinking it would give me a constant reminder that I have diabetes," recalls Rebecca Sneider, 28, of Brookline, Massachusetts. However, she quickly got used to it. "If anything, it's a reminder in a good way because I've been feeling better."

Who's a Candidate for the Pump?

It used to be that diabetes care professionals would recommend the pump only to certain types of patients:

- People who experience the dawn phenomenon—early morning elevations in blood glucose, probably caused by the release of certain hormones at night. (Pump users can compensate for the dawn phenomenon by programming a higher basal infusion rate in the early morning.)
- Women who are pregnant or thinking about becoming pregnant, who must strive for excellent blood glucose control as early as possible in the pregnancy.
- People with hectic lifestyles that could undermine good control over blood sugar levels with rigid insulin injection schedules.
- People who have been unable to adequately control their blood glucose levels using MDI.

These indications are changing and broadening. Howard Wolpert, M.D., senior physician and the director of the Insulin Pump Program at the Joslin Diabetes Center in Boston, is convinced that pumps can be especially beneficial to people with frequent episodes of severe hypoglycemia.

"If you go back about 10 years, the use of a pump in someone with frequent hypoglycemia and hypoglycemia unawareness was absolutely contraindicated, the concern being that pump therapy would exacerbate the problem," he says. "But it's clear that in a certain subset of patients, pumps can actually provide more stable insulin delivery, reduce the blood sugar fluctuations, and actually minimize hypoglycemia."

For years, George Owen, 40, of Duxbury, Massachusetts, had been battling bouts of hypoglycemia without warning, losing consciousness more often than he'd like to remember. He and his wife worked at the same office. When he left to become a freelance consultant, his wife became concerned that no one would be around to seek medical attention for his blackouts. Since going on the pump two years ago, he's had fewer episodes. "I do have one every once in a while," he says. "But it's been a dramatic improvement."

As diabetes professionals have redefined what defines "good control," more and more people with Type 1 diabetes have become potential candidates for pump therapy. Usually, the best candidates are those already familiar with intensive insulin therapy who are using MDI and frequent blood glucose monitoring. They know how to troubleshoot when things don't go according to plan. And they're team players, working with their healthcare professionals.

"I always listen to people's expectations," says Virginia Peragallo-Dittko, R.N., C.D.E., a diabetes nurse specialist at Winthrop-University Hospital in Mineola, New York. "Some people think this is just going to remove all of the burdens of managing diabetes—and it doesn't."

Farkas-Hirsch concurs, "People who are not willing to go through the educational process and carry out all the aspects of an intensive management program are probably not the best candidates," she says. "You can't just hook on the pump and expect good things to happen. You don't get 'fixed' with a pump."

Unfortunately, she says, some people do manage to get hold of pumps without ever getting the proper education. Sometimes they wind up with severe hypoglycemia or diabetic ketoacidosis because they never learned how to balance their bolus rates with their carbohydrate intake. Worse yet, they don't always learn to recognize the symptoms and wait to seek help until they're in real trouble—and land in the emergency room. "Sometimes they're lucky and sort of do all right, but we've also seen some real disasters where people have gotten into serious problems with pumps because they didn't get all the information they needed," she says.

Insulin pumps aren't cheap by any stretch of the imagination. The pumps themselves cost about $5,000 to $5,500, and the basic supplies can run up to $150 a month. So, when considering pump therapy, it is important to take cost into consideration. . . .

Using an Insulin Analog

Lispro (brand name Humalog), an insulin analog that works even faster than regular insulin, was first used in injection regimens to cover the mealtime rise in blood sugar, but increasingly it is used in insulin pumps. When used in pumps Lispro appears to offer even better control than regular insulin, when used in pumps. Not unexpectedly, it's better suited to mealtime boluses, but it is also better for basal infusion, according to Bernard Zinman, M.D., director of the Banting and Best Diabetes Center at the University of Toronto in Canada.

"When you're adjusting basal rates, changing the basal infusion rate translates more quickly into a change in circulating insulin levels when you're using Lispro compared with human regular insulin," says Dr. Zinman. "Thus, the desired metabolic response is achieved more effectively."

In 1997, Dr. Zinman and colleagues published a study in the journal *Diabetes* comparing the use of human regular insulin and Lispro in pumps. Results from the study showed that those using Lispro had lower hemoglobin A1c levels (a test that shows average blood sugar levels over the previous three months) as well as a reduced risk of hypoglycemia. The biggest disadvantage of Lispro in pumps is that, if the infusion rate should get interrupted, people using Lispro will become insulin deficient more quickly and may develop hyperglycemia and ketoacidosis more rapidly.

Fortunately, the newer pumps are more reliable and have alarms to alert the user of interrupted insulin flow, so this risk should be minimal, according to Dr. Zinman. "It isn't something to be terribly concerned about, but it's something people should be aware of when they're using Lispro in their pumps."

Use in pumps is not an FDA-approved indication for Lispro, but many doctors are already going ahead and prescribing it "off label." By pump manufacturers' estimates, at least 75 percent of Disetronic pump users and 80 percent of MiniMed pump users currently infuse Lispro.

The Future of Pumps

"What we're really shooting for is a 'closed-loop' insulin delivery system in which an implantable glucose sensor continuously measures blood glucose, passes the information on to an implantable insulin pump, and the pump responds to the information by modifying its insulin output accordingly," says Christopher Saudek, M.D., professor of medicine and director of the Johns Hopkins Diabetes Center at the Johns Hopkins School of Medicine in Baltimore.

How likely is such an "artificial pancreas" to become a reality? Already, some of the pieces are in place.

Implantable insulin pumps have been used in hundreds of patients worldwide in research settings since the mid-1980s. The disc-shaped pump, which is about 3.5 inches in diameter, is implanted into the abdomen in a minor surgical operation similar to implanting a cardiac pacemaker. The implanted pump infuses insulin into the peritoneal cavity, and users can control the infusion rates using a remote-control device. The pump has a special reservoir that must be refilled with U400 insulin (four times as strong as the insulin commonly used for insulin injections) every three months or so using a special syringe.

According to Dr. Saudek, the advantages to these pumps are that they stay in place, are cosmetically acceptable, and would make users less susceptible to infection than externally worn pumps do. The insulin these pumps deliver goes preferentially to the liver—just like insulin from a healthy pancreas does—which is thought to provide better blood sugar control with less hypoglycemia.

One of the most serious complications of implantable pumps has been catheter blockage, but reformulation of the insulin used in implantable pumps has largely eliminated this problem. MiniMed Technologies' implantable pumps are now cleared for marketing in Europe and the company plans to apply soon for FDA approval to market them in the United States.

A closed-loop system would also include an implantable sensor that would continuously monitor glucose levels. A number of biotech companies have unveiled designs for continuous monitoring systems and are working toward FDA approval for marketing the monitors to consumers in the United States.

Dr. Saudek says he's confident that the closed-loop system will someday become a reality, but says it's difficult to estimate how long it will take. "I do believe young people now with Type 1 diabetes will be around to see it," he asserts.

THE PROMISE OF ISLET TRANSPLANTATION

Roger Doughty

Theoretically, the transplantation of healthy islet cells that produce insulin could mean a cure for diabetes, writes Roger Doughty in the following selection. Doughty explains, however, that actual islet transplants have had limited success because few of the fragile cells survive the transfer and the body rejects the foreign cells. In addition, he notes, antirejection drugs often have severe side effects. Nevertheless, Doughty observes, because islet transplants would ultimately be cheaper and less invasive than pancreas transplants, researchers are looking for ways to make islet transplantation more successful. For example, pig islets encased in gel capsules cured diabetic monkeys for over two years, the author reports, and other researchers have had success with new drugs that prevent the immune system from attacking the foreign islets. Islet transplant technology is improving, says Doughty, and some patients are remaining insulin free for longer periods. Although the islets eventually stop functioning, most patients claim the attempt was worth it. Doughty is a freelance writer and frequent contributor to *Diabetes Forecast*, a publication of the American Diabetes Association.

Ever since Mary Shelley crafted her classic tale of Dr. Frankenstein and his manufactured monster, fiction writers, moviemakers, and TV producers have fascinated us with stories about creatures with bionic limbs and multiple brains. In comparison, transplanting an organ—or cells—from one person to another seems pretty simple.

Not quite, says Paul Gores, MD, director of pancreas and islet transplantation at the Carolinas Medical Center in Charlotte, and one of the nation's leading organ transplanters. While Gores concedes that solid organ transplants—kidneys, hearts, livers, even pancreases—are now considered routine, he says we still have a way to go before cellular transplants make it into that category. That's because the endocrine system cells, which include pancreatic islet cells, are so fragile.

Looking for a Cure

Transplanting live islet cells, in theory, would "cure" diabetes. For example, it should be possible to transplant healthy islet cells into a newly diagnosed child, eliminating diabetes before it has a chance to do any long-term damage. With approximately 30,000 new cases of type 1 diabetes reported in the United States alone each year, the idea of enlisting the aid of islets to stop the disease dead in its tracks has widespread appeal.

Since 1893, when surgeons in Bristol, England, transplanted part of a sheep's pancreas into a human (the patient died from infection), doctors have been fascinated by the prospect of making islets live up to their potential. So far the cells have been less than cooperative, despite the expenditure of tens of millions of dollars to find ways to make them get their act together.

What medical science has been able to offer so far is an experimental procedure that no physician would dream of attempting on a child, or even on most adults. But based on a number of innovative developments in the area of pancreatic islet cell transplantation, there's renewed hope that someday, not too far down the road, theory will become reality. "There's a lot of impressive data out there, and this is a hot area again," says the Carolina surgeon. "Everyone in the field is feeling optimistic."

What excites Gores is the arrival of new and more effective antirejection drugs as well as the knowledge that his colleagues around the country and abroad are working simultaneously on a variety of techniques to perfect the tricky business of transplanting islets.

Surgeons and scientists feel they've found ways to transplant islet cells alone, without piggybacking on a whole organ transplant (the previous requirement); others have set out to prove that islet cells removed from pigs might be as good as human islets for transplanting; some are experimenting with membrane capsules designed to protect islets from the ravaging attacks of the body's immune system, giving them a better chance to establish themselves and function. To add to the mix, a bunch of monkeys in Miami that used to have diabetes, but don't any longer, are making headline news.

As exciting as these and other studies sound, Gores counsels caution. "We want to avoid getting people's hopes too high that anything we're doing will result in an instant cure for diabetes," he warns. "We've seen that happen too many times before."

Gores is all too familiar with the hype that has surrounded islet cell transplantation in the past. "I used to have a slide I used as part of a talk," he recalls. "It's the cover story from a medical publication that came out in 1975. The headline says, 'Islet Cell Transplantation: The Cure for Diabetes Is Just Around the Corner.' People have been exposed to that kind of misinformation for years."

Understanding the Basics

There are about one million islets in a human pancreas, which is located in the center of the abdomen, right underneath the stomach. The islets make up only about 2 percent of the pancreas. Beta cells, the ones that produce insulin, make up 75 to 80 percent of the islets. The rest of the pancreatic cells produce enzymes to help digest food, which are discharged into the intestines.

Healthy beta cells release enough insulin to maintain normal glucose levels in the body. When they fall victim to the body's immune system and fail to function, diabetes results.

Surgeons in New York may have attempted the first islet transplant in conjunction with a kidney transplant way back in 1935. (After 65 years the documentation is a bit sketchy.) It's a matter of record that Minnesota transplanters attempted the islet-kidney procedure in 1974. From that time on, the public has been titillated by stories depicting an islet-induced "cure" for diabetes. But the cure has remained elusive.

The problem lies with the beta cells themselves; as noted previously, they are extremely fragile. It's been estimated that only about half survive the trip from the scene of their removal to the transplant site. Half of those survivors probably die before being injected. It's likely that only 25 percent of those transplanted engraft in the recipient's body.

The body's immune system, which has no way of knowing the transplanted cells are trying to be helpful, launches attacks against them. The drugs used to prevent rejection, especially cyclosporine and prednisone, compound the problem by impairing the ability of the new islets to respond to glucose and produce insulin and by the severe side effects they can cause, including life-threatening infections and cancer. Because of these factors and technical glitches, islet cell transplantation has failed to live up to the hopes and dreams of the surgeons, transplant immunologists, diabetologists, cell biologists, and engineers who have worked so hard to perfect it.

Why Not Transplant Pancreases?

Since a non-insulin-producing pancreas is the culprit, the most obvious solution would be to give every person with type 1 diabetes, particularly every newly diagnosed person, a pancreas transplant and be done with it. The procedure's success rate has climbed this past decade, (82–86 percent when kidneys are transplanted along with a pancreas, which is the most common method; somewhat lower, 62–74 percent, with pancreas-only transplants), even though the organ recipients often have already encountered major diabetes complications. And, theoretically, there are enough pancreases to go around.

David E.R. Sutherland, MD, director of the Diabetes Institute for

Immunology and Transplantation at the University of Minnesota, says that of the approximately 5,000 cadaver donors in the United States each year, only about 1,500 of the pancreases are used for transplants. He estimates that at least 3,000 suitable pancreases are available each year and says that thanks to techniques that make dividing the pancreas in half possible (in 1979, Sutherland performed the world's first living-donor half-pancreas transplant), 6,000 transplants could be performed from cadaver donors.

"There were 3,000 living kidney donors in the United States in 1996," says the surgeon. "If we had 3,000 living pancreas donors we could do nearly 10,000 pancreas transplants per year in the United States, making it possible for one-third of the patients with new-onset diabetes to have one."

While Sutherland's math is on the mark, he acknowledges that most patients, given a choice, would prefer a less invasive islet procedure, if it worked, to the trauma of major surgery. "Islet transplants will replace pancreas transplants," he says. "I think eventually pancreas programs will be obsolete."

Pancreas transplants can be pricey, too, with hospitalization and physician fees running up to $100,000 and immunosuppressive drugs (with potential serious side effects) costing from $5,000 to $20,000 a year in some cases. However, pancreas transplants are often covered by medical insurance, and Medicare coverage for the procedure became available in 1999.

Reducing the Cost of Diabetes

In contrast, islet cell transplants, which cost between $75,000 and $100,000, aren't covered by medical insurance.

Bernhard Hering, MD, director of the University of Minnesota's islet cell transplant program, predicts that the bottom line will eventually convince health insurance companies to pick up the cost of islet cell transplants.

"The total lifetime cost for type 1 diabetes could be reduced from $600,000 to around $100,000 if islet transplant becomes available without the need for immunosuppressive treatment," Hering reasons. "The health insurance industry will benefit from what we are doing."

Much of Hering's optimism stems from the formation in October 1999 of the Collaborative Network for Clinical Research on Immune Tolerance. The 40 network centers, which will conduct trials of "tolergenic" drugs, are located in the United States, Canada, Germany, Italy, and Australia. "Sharing our knowledge and expertise increases our chances of achieving success more quickly," says Hering. "I believe that the year 2000 will mark a turning point in the history of islet cell transplantation."

One of those "tolergenic" drugs worked well on the Miami monkeys (six to be exact), which have stayed insulin free for more than a year after receiving islet cell transplants. The monkeys don't need immunosuppressive drugs, either. Monthly shots of anti-CD 154, a new immune system modulator made by Biogen, Inc., seem to be doing the trick. Human trials using anti-CD 154 began in the summer of 1999, but were halted in October 1999 because of clotting side effects observed in trials not related to islet cell transplantation.

Camillo Ricordi, MD, who heads up the Diabetes Research Institute at the University of Miami, home of the monkeys, says he's concerned about the delay in the trial, but confident the manufacturer will solve the problem. "Anti-CD 154 is the best agent we've tested so far," says Ricordi, "and we haven't observed any problems in association with islet cell transplantation. But we agree that patient safety must be an absolute priority, so we'll just have to wait. My belief is that we'll get the OK to resume trials by the middle of 2000."

Ricordi and Hering point to rapamycin as another drug with great potential. Although rapamycin is an immunosuppressant, it can be combined with other drugs in a "synergistic regimen" to induce tolerance. That allows doctors to reduce the use of cyclosporine and prednisone by up to 50 percent. Trials involving rapamycin in combination with various other drugs are under way at several locations. Anti IL-2 receptor antibody, another promising antirejection drug, is also being tested in Miami.

Hering is looking forward to the day when islet cell transplants will be performed on an outpatient basis. "We want to make the procedure simple and convenient," he says. He foresees a future in which injected islet transplantation will lead to "patients coming in once a month for a follow-up injection of antibodies that will keep them insulin free for the rest of their lives. The most promising transplant method being explored is similar to an intravenous drip, which isn't considered to be a major medical procedure. The islets are dripped into the liver, where they take hold and begin to function on their own.

"Circumventing the need for chronic immunosuppressive therapy, which it appears likely we'll be able to do with the new drugs we have, will greatly lower the cost for endocrine cell replacement therapy in the future," predicts Hering.

Bring in the Pigs

The dog's reign as man's best friend may be in jeopardy, at least if the man (or woman) in question happens to be a medical researcher. His or her preference would probably be the pig.

Pharmaceutical and medical device companies have been breeding pigs and raising their offspring in sterile sites for years, and certain pig tissues, such as skin and heart valves, have already been used in humans. Pigs can be bred rapidly and raised free of known diseases.

While barnyard porkers are unsuitable for transplant purposes, today's high tech pigs are prepared for the task before they ever see the light of day, the result of human DNA being inserted into fertilized pig eggs. These super swine produce both human and porcine proteins. Best of all, islets from the "improved" pigs secrete humanlike insulin. Breeders have invested millions in the hope that the islets, hearts, livers, kidneys, lungs, and pancreases of these special pigs will prove to be just what the doctors ordered.

Progress on the pig front has been promising. In 1996, Anthony M. Sun, MD, of the University of Toronto, reported that he and his team had successfully cured monkeys with diabetes for up to 802 days without immunosuppression using transplanted pig islets encased in gel capsules. Gores cautions that these results concern monkeys only—it's possible that the process would not work in humans.

Used in the delivery of everything from hormone replacement to time-released medication, encapsulation has long been seen as a way to protect islets from attack by the immune system while allowing them to secrete insulin and receive the nutrients and oxygen they need to survive. While sphere-like microbeads have been the norm, scientists at Miami's Diabetes Research Institute, home of the monkeys, are experimenting with alternate shapes, including spaghetti-like strands.

Keeping an Eye on Islets

Hering, who established and coordinates the International Islet Transplant Registry, in addition to being the associate director of Minnesota's Diabetes Institute for Immunology and Transplantation, says that of the 375 islet cell transplants performed at 35 institutions worldwide from 1974 through 1999 (all in conjunction with whole organ transplants) only 45 resulted in the recipients becoming insulin independent for more than one week. (One recipient did remain insulin free for more than five years.) Eventually, however, the islets stop functioning and the recipients must resume taking insulin shots.

The vast majority of islet transplants have taken place in the United States, while 60 were performed in Germany and 30 in Italy.

Gores, who performed two successful islet cell transplants in 1993 (one patient stayed insulin free for 18 months), sums up the frustration of fighting so many losing battles with the immune system. "With such a minute success ratio," he says, "it's easy to understand why people got discouraged."

Still, as Hering points out, when islet transplants don't succeed, they're rarely complete failures. Patients usually experience dramatic reductions in the amount of insulin they must inject, some for years, and insulin reactions are greatly reduced. Most say it was worth a try. "Another good thing," observes Hering, "is that it isn't fatal. If a heart or liver transplant fails, the patient could die. If an islet transplant fails, the patient can still inject insulin and the possibility of trying again exists."

As recently as 1995 even devout islet advocates appeared ready to throw in the towel and move on to other projects. More effective anti-rejection drugs, sorely needed to achieve better outcomes, seemed stalled in the pipeline; investors walked away from several projects seen as promising but unprofitable; and a highly publicized pig islet encapsulation technique researched by Patrick Soon Shiong, MD, proved to be ineffective.

The picture brightened in 1996 when Hering, then working at Justus-Liebig-University of Giessen in his native Germany, caught the transplant world's attention by heading up a protocol that concluded with nine of 12 patients maintaining graft function for more than one year. Four became insulin-independent. He credits an increase in the number of islets engrafted and a reduction in the use of steroids as part of the immunosuppressive treatment as key factors.

According to Hering, islet cell transplanters have three goals. "The first is to match the 80 percent success rate of a pancreas transplant without the need for surgery. The second is to eliminate the need for continued use of immunosuppressive drugs, and the third is to make islet cell transplantation routine and available to children. Today we have the tools we need. All we have to do is learn how to use them effectively."

Hering says it's now possible to increase the number of islet cells that engraft to 50 to 60 percent. That, coupled with the advent of anti-CD 154, rapamycin, which can induce tolerance before a transplant, and anti IL-2 receptor antibody, leads him to believe that medical science is finally on the brink of a breakthrough. "I believe there could be as many as 300 islet cell transplants this year, with a success ratio of 50 percent or higher. That would generate enormous momentum and enthusiasm.

"Transplanters didn't contribute much to this," says Hering. "The only thing that has really changed is that immunology has advanced. The immunosuppressive drugs we've been using are so toxic that 20 percent of non-diabetic patients who receive kidney transplants eventually develop diabetes as a result of taking the drugs. They replace one disease with another. These new drugs no longer cause diabetes and may be very effective in preventing rejection.". . .

A Spirit of Cooperation

While everyone would love to be the first to find the illusive cure, a sense of cooperation rather than competition prevails in the islet transplant community. The one-for-all and all-for-one attitude displayed by those waging war against diabetes has become a force to be reckoned with.

"There are many options being explored right now," says Minnesota's Hering. "Maybe we can combine some, or find more than one answer. Perhaps the day will come when, rather than worrying about how to solve the problem, we can offer patients some choices."

That day can't come too soon for the intrepid islet investigators. All are motivated, some for personal reasons.

North Carolina's Gores is haunted by the memory of a former patient who gained insulin-independence after her islet transplant in 1993 and delighted in a life of lower insulin doses. Then the islets finally failed.

"I used to hear from her every Christmas," the surgeon recalls. "She'd bring me up to date on what was going on in her life. I didn't think too much about it when I didn't hear anything a few years ago. I thought something came up and she just didn't get around to contacting me. Later I heard from a nurse that she had died from an unrelated illness that April.

"When I think about her life I get discouraged. She was diagnosed at the age of three and didn't receive her islet transplant until she was 31. So she spent most of her life battling diabetes and only got to fully enjoy the last few years. That just isn't good enough. Until we can intervene in a child's life at three, bring diabetes to an end, and let that child make the most of his or her life, our work won't be done."

Alternative Treatment of Diabetes with Natural Therapeutics

Alan R. Gaby and Trina M. Seligman

Alternative treatments have been shown to provide diabetics with safer, more effective methods of maintaining blood glucose levels and minimizing the adverse effects of diabetes, write Alan R. Gaby and Trina M. Seligman. In the following selection, the authors review research that shows the effectiveness of alternative dietary regimens, nutritional supplements, and herbal treatments. For example, a high-fiber diet reduced the need for insulin in some diabetics, and chromium supplements improved glucose tolerance. The authors also explain that diabetics who maintain normal blood glucose levels according to conventional therapy still exhibit complications as a result of other metabolic abnormalities. These pathological changes can be minimized using alternative methods, including vitamin C, which inhibits some of the biochemical processes that result in diabetic complications, and vitamin B-12, which has been used to successfully treat diabetic eye disease. Gaby is an expert in nutritional therapies and a professor of nutrition at Bastyr University in Seattle, Washington. Seligman practices at Evergreen Integrative Medicine.

Diabetes is a chronic disease characterized by elevated blood glucose levels and disturbances in carbohydrate, fat and protein metabolism. These metabolic abnormalities result in part from a deficiency of the blood sugar–lowering hormone insulin or from "insulin resistance" (a defect in the body's capacity to respond to insulin).

Type 1 diabetes, also known as insulin-dependent diabetes mellitus (IDDM), usually begins in childhood and is thought to be a result of autoimmune destruction of the pancreatic beta cells (the cells that produce insulin; also called islet cells). Destruction of the beta cells results in complete or almost-complete loss of insulin production, thereby necessitating insulin injections to maintain blood sugar control.

Type 2 diabetes, also known as non-insulin-dependent diabetes mellitus (NIDDM), is usually diagnosed after 40 years of age. Type 2 diabetes is frequently associated with insulin resistance and normal or even elevated levels of insulin, although subnormal insulin levels are also seen in some type 2 diabetics.

Gestational diabetes is characterized by hyperglycemia (elevated blood sugar) during pregnancy and usually disappears after the child is delivered. However, even though gestational diabetes may be relatively short-lived, it can compromise the health of both mother and fetus.

Diabetes is associated with a number of significant medical problems.

- Severe hyperglycemia may result in coma or even death. Milder hyperglycemia, if present for many years, increases the risk of cardiovascular disease, which can manifest as a heart attack, congestive heart failure, stroke, gangrene of the extremities (necessitating amputation in some cases), or kidney failure.
- Atherosclerosis [narrowing and hardening of the arteries] accounts for up to 60% of all diabetes-related deaths.
- In addition, as many as 33% of all cases of kidney dialysis and 50% of all amputations in the United States and Europe are a result of complications from diabetes.
- Individuals with diabetes are 2-to-20 times more likely to develop cardiovascular disease or stroke than are people without diabetes.
- Visual loss due to retinopathy (damage to the retina of the eye) or cataract is also common among diabetics. In fact, diabetes is the leading cause of blindness among American adults between ages 20 and 74 years, and is responsible for as many as 40,000 new cases of blindness annually in the United States.
- Neuropathy (nerve damage) occurs in about half of all diabetics during the course of their disease.
- Diabetics also tend to suffer from poor wound healing and impaired immune function.

The Conventional Approach

It is now well accepted that maintaining blood glucose levels as close to the normal range as possible will reduce the incidence of these complications. Conventional physicians attempt to regulate blood glucose through a combination of dietary modification, weight loss when appropriate, exercise, and blood sugar–lowering medications, including insulin and so-called "oral hypoglycemic agents." Although this approach is helpful to some extent, it has limitations. First, the conventional dietary approach often fails to emphasize high-fiber, high-complex-carbohydrate foods, or specific foods such as legumes, which have been shown to improve glycemic (blood glucose) control. Consequently, the standard "diabetic diet" is frequently not as effective as it could be. Furthermore, insulin therapy may not achieve satisfactory glycemic control in patients with insulin resistance, and oral hypoglycemic [blood sugar–lowering] agents may lose their efficacy after five or more years of treatment. When these drugs are effective, they must be used with caution, because an excessive dose can cause medically significant hypoglycemia. For these and other reasons, the conventional treatment of diabetes often produces less-than-adequate blood glucose control. In addition, insulin itself is believed to be a cause of cardiovascular disease, so safer methods of lowering blood glucose are urgently needed.

It should be noted that the blood glucose concentration is not the only determinant of diabetic end-organ damage (i.e., neuropathy, retinopathy, nephropathy [kidney damage], etc.). Diabetic complications still occur (albeit with a lower frequency) in patients who carefully maintain their blood sugar near or even completely within the normal range. A number of metabolic abnormalities and pathological changes that are associated with diabetes may be at least partly independent of blood sugar levels. These include increased production of oxygen-derived free radicals, excessive platelet aggregation and protein glycosylation, and intracellular accumulation of sorbitol. Although these abnormalities are not fully understood, it is possible that taking measures to correct them will help prevent some of the complications of diabetes.

Other Determinants of Diabetic Complications

Oxygen-derived free radicals are normal by-products of metabolism. However, these compounds are highly reactive and can cause significant damage (often called oxidative damage) to cell membranes and other cellular structures. Free-radical damage is believed to play a role in atherosclerosis, cataract formation, and some of the other complications of diabetes. To counteract the destructiveness of free radicals, the body possesses a complex system of antioxidant defenses that utilize various vitamins, minerals, and other naturally occurring substances. Diabetics have been reported to have significantly higher free-radical activity, as well as significantly lower concentrations of antioxidants, compared with healthy controls. These changes were of greater magnitude in patients with disease complications than in those without complications. It is possible, therefore, that supplementing with foods, nutrients, and herbs that have antioxidant activity would help prevent diabetic end-organ damage.

Another factor that contributes to the complications of diabetes is a process called glycosylation of proteins. Known to chemists as the Maillard reaction and to bakers as the browning reaction, glycosylation involves the irreversible binding of glucose or other sugars to a protein molecule. A growing body of evidence indicates that glycosylation of tissue proteins is one of the mechanisms whereby diabetics develop organ damage. Although glycosylation occurs continuously in all human beings, the reaction is accelerated when blood sugar is elevated. One of the reasons that maintaining tight blood sugar control prevents complications is that the rate of tissue glycosylation is lower when the average blood sugar is lower. However, studies have shown that certain nutritional supplements also inhibit glycosylation independently of any effect they may have on blood glucose levels. Supplementation with these nutrients might therefore be expected to reduce the risk of diabetic end-organ damage.

Another process that leads to diabetes-related organ damage is the accumulation of sorbitol in certain tissues and organs. Sorbitol is manufactured in the body from glucose. When glucose levels are elevated, sorbitol is produced inside the cells faster than it can be broken down. Since sorbitol cannot cross cell membranes, it builds up inside the cells and draws water in by the process of osmosis. This sorbitol-induced osmotic swelling is believed to be one of the main causes of tissue damage in diabetics.

Glucose is converted to sorbitol by the enzyme aldose reductase. A drug called sorbinil, which inhibits this enzyme, was shown to reverse both diabetic neuropathy and diabetic cataracts. However, because of its severe toxicity, sorbinil was rejected by the Food and Drug Administration for use as a prescription drug. Substances which can safely prevent the accumulation of intracellular sorbitol would therefore be welcome.

Alternative Strategies for Treating Diabetes

The above evidence suggests that appropriate goals in the management of diabetes include maintaining blood glucose levels as close to the normal range as possible, minimizing the adverse effects of free radicals by enhancing antioxidant defenses, and reducing the glycosylation of proteins and the intracellular accumulation of sorbitol. A number of different interventions that are currently considered to be in the realm of "alternative medicine" have been shown to accomplish one or more of these goals. In addition, specific methods of preventing or treating diabetic complications (such as cardiovascular disease and neuropathy) have been identified.

A considerable body of evidence indicates that a diet high in fiber and complex carbohydrates helps improve glucose regulation in diabetics. In one study, 20 insulin-treated diabetics who were not overweight consumed a standard diabetic diet (providing 43% of calories as carbohydrate) for seven days, followed by a high-complex-carbohydrate, high fiber (HCF) diet for 16 days. The HCF diet provided approximately 70% of calories as carbohydrate and was designed to maintain body weight. The daily dose of insulin was lower for each patient on the HCF diet than on the control diet and the mean insulin dose was reduced significantly from 26 to 11 units/day. On the HCF diet, insulin therapy could be discontinued in nine patients who had been receiving 15–20 units per day and in two patients who had been receiving 32 units per day. Blood glucose levels in the fasting state and three hours after meals were lower in most patients on the HCF diet, even though the insulin dose had been reduced. The mean serum cholesterol concentration also fell significantly from 206 to 147 milligrams per deciliter (mg/dl). This study demonstrates that a HCF diet can reduce blood sugar levels and insulin requirements in diabetics and that this effect is not dependent on weight loss. In a follow-up study, the beneficial effects of this diet were maintained for periods ranging from 26 to 86 months. A HCF diet has also been found to reduce insulin requirements in patients with type 1 diabetes.

In another study, 16 diabetics consumed a conventional carbohydrate-restricted diet or a diet which excluded refined carbohydrate but allowed unrefined carbohydrate. On the unrefined-carbohydrate diet, the mean postprandial (after-meal) plasma glucose concentration fell significantly by 20%. Supplementation with 78 grams per day (g/day) of wheat bran has also been shown to reduce the insulin requirements of insulin-dependent diabetics by 8–10%.

Ingestion of legumes appears to be particularly effective at controlling blood sugar. Eighteen non-insulin-dependent diabetics and nine insulin-dependent diabetics received a high-complex-carbohydrate diet containing leguminous fiber, and a standard low-carbohydrate diet, each for six weeks, in random order. In both groups, the mean concentrations of blood glucose (preprandial and 2-hour postprandial) and serum cholesterol, and the urinary excretion of glucose were all significantly lower on the diet containing legumes than on the standard diet. In another study, breakfasts containing lentils or wholemeal bread of identical carbohydrate content were consumed by seven healthy volunteers. Compared with bread, the lentils produced a significant 71% reduction in the area under the blood glucose curve and flattened the plasma insulin response. These changes are indicative of improved glucose metabolism. In addition, the lentil breakfast lowered the blood glucose response to a standard bread lunch four hours later. This study demonstrates that the beneficial effect of legumes on glucose control extends to the meal after which they are consumed.

The Impact of Certain Foods

Certain individual foods have also been shown to lower blood glucose or to improve carbohydrate tolerance in diabetics. Ingestion of 100 g/day of whole barley flour for four weeks by healthy volunteers significantly reduced the blood-glucose response to a test meal (bread). In another study, addition of 600 g/day of green beans or 60 g/day of fresh onions to the diet for one week significantly lowered blood sugar levels in a group of patients with poorly controlled diabetes. Ingestion of an onion extract has also been shown to reduce the rise in blood sugar in healthy volunteers during a glucose tolerance test. Both garlic and onions reduced the hyperglycemic effect of glucose feeding in experimental animals.

The inclusion of garlic and onions in the diet of diabetics may be desirable for reasons other than their potential to lower blood glucose. Garlic has been reported to decrease serum cholesterol levels, to prevent the oxidation of LDL cholesterol, to inhibit platelet aggregation, and to lower blood pressure. Each of these effects would be expected to prevent the development of disease, one of the most important complications of diabetes. Onion extracts have also been shown to inhibit platelet aggregation and to lower blood pressure in patients with hypertension. In addition, onions contain relatively large amounts of quercetin, a flavonoid compound that inhibits aldose reductase. Since aldose reductase inhibition has been shown to reverse diabetic cataracts and neuropathy, inclusion of onions in the diet of diabetics seems desirable. Brewer's yeast may also be useful for diabetics, as it has been reported to contain at least two blood sugar–lowering compounds. The capacity of yeast to reduce blood glucose was reported as early as 1923, although the type of yeast used was not specified in that report.

Twenty-one patients with diabetic neuropathy consumed a vegan diet (free of meat, chicken, fish, eggs, and dairy products) consisting of unrefined foods; these patients also participated in an exercise program. In 17 of the 21 cases, the sharp, stabbing, shooting, and/or burning pains were completely alleviated within 4–16 days. Numbness persisted, but was noticeably improved within two days. The improvement in diabetic neuropathy did not appear to be a result of better blood glucose control.

Epidemiologic studies have found an increased risk of type 1 diabetes among children who consumed cow's milk early in life. It has been postulated that ingestion of cow's milk results in the production of antibodies that cross-react with and damage pancreatic insulin-producing cells. However, other studies have found no association between ingestion of cow's milk and the risk of developing type 1 diabetes. Further research is needed to resolve the conflicting data.

The Role of Nutritional Supplements

Glucose regulation depends on a wide range of vitamins, minerals, and other micronutrients. Many of these nutrients are in short supply in the typical refined, processed American diet. In addition, some nutrients have been shown to exert effects that might be expected to reduce the risk of end-organ damage. Supplementation with appropriate vitamins and minerals may therefore be of value in the prevention and treatment of diabetes. Following is a review of specific nutrients:

Chromium is a component of a molecule called glucose-tolerance factor (GTF), which occurs naturally in the body and enhances the action of insulin at the cellular level. Rats fed a chromium-deficient diet developed hyperglycemia and glycosuria. Monkeys maintained on a low-chromium diet had abnormal glucose metabolism, which was corrected by chromium supplementation. Chromium also protected guinea pigs against experimentally induced pancreatic beta-cell destruction and reduced insulin resistance in genetically obese mice.

Chromium deficiency is known to occur in man. Individuals maintained on parenteral nutrition developed a complex metabolic disorder including impaired glucose tolerance, which was reversed by chromium supplementation. Less severe forms of chromium deficiency may be common in the United States. Because of farming techniques which fail to replenish trace minerals in the soil, the chromium content of food is probably lower than it was at the turn of the century. Tissue chromium levels were found to decline with age in Americans, but not in individuals living in other countries. One dietary survey revealed that 90% of American diets contained less than the minimum suggested daily intake for chromium.

In a double-blind trial, daily administration of 200 micrograms (mcg) of chromium produced a significant reduction in 2-hour postprandial glucose levels in elderly women with borderline glucose tolerance. In another study of elderly patients, chromium supplementation significantly reduced plasma glucose concentrations during a glucose tolerance test and significantly improved glucose utilization. Treatment with 150 mcg/day of chromium for four months normalized glucose tolerance in four of ten elderly individuals with abnormal glucose tolerance. Administration of 150 to 1,000 mcg/day of chromium improved glucose tolerance in three of six diabetics. The larger doses were more effective than the smaller doses.

Other studies have produced negative results. In two double-blind studies, supplementation with 150 or 200 mcg/day of chromium failed to improve glucose tolerance in diabetic patients. These conflicting results may be due to several factors. First, in all of the studies described above, chromium chloride was used. Because absorption of this form of chromium is only about 0.5%, the dosage may have been inadequate. Second, in order to exert an effect on glucose metabolism, inorganic chromium must be converted to GTF. Biosynthesis of GTF requires, among other things, an adequate supply of niacin, a nutrient which may be in short supply in many individuals.

Ingestion of foods containing GTF may therefore be a preferred way of obtaining biologically active chromium. GTF occurs naturally in brewer's yeast and to a lesser extent in other foods, including beef, chicken, bananas, lobster, shrimp, mushrooms, and cheese. GTF chromium is also promoted as a nutritional supplement. However, according to W. Mertz, who originally discovered GTF, analysis of one of the so-called "GTF chromium" products revealed no GTF activity. The exact molecular structure of GTF is still unknown, and no one has been able to synthesize it. Therefore, claims that "GTF chromium" supplements are superior to other well-absorbed forms of chromium (such as chromium aspartate, chromium picolinate, or chromium polynicotinate) are questionable.

The Impact of Niacin and Niacinamide

As a component of GTF, niacin (nicotinic acid) plays an important role in carbohydrate metabolism. Many refined foods consumed by Americans are depleted of niacin. Grains and other foods that are "enriched" usually contain added niacinamide, which is capable of performing most of the functions of Vitamin B3, but which cannot apparently be converted by the human body into niacin. In addition, most vitamin supplements contain niacinamide rather than niacin. A small amount of niacin may therefore be necessary for some individuals to enable the production of adequate amounts of GTF.

In one study, 16 healthy elderly individuals received either 200 mcg of chromium, 100 mg of niacin, or both, daily for 28 days. Fasting plasma glucose levels and glucose tolerance were not affected by either chromium or niacin individually. However, the combination of chromium plus niacin produced a significant 14.8% decrease in the area under the glucose curve during a glucose tolerance test and a significant 6.8% reduction in fasting glucose. This study suggests that a relatively low dose of supplemental niacin, when combined with chromium, improves glucose metabolism and may therefore be useful for preventing and treating diabetes.

Larger doses of niacin (such as 1–3 g/day) can effectively lower serum cholesterol levels and reduce the risk of cardiovascular disease. Although this treatment is often prescribed by conventional physicians, many doctors are reluctant to recommend high-dose niacin for hypercholesterolemic diabetics because it will occasionally increase blood glucose levels in diabetics. However, the effect of high-dose niacin is variable and this vitamin has also been reported to reduce insulin requirements in some type 1 diabetics. Consequently, high-dose niacin is not contraindicated in diabetics; however, blood glucose levels should be monitored closely.

Both niacin and niacinamide may also help prevent the onset or progression of diabetes by protecting the insulin-producing pancreatic beta cells from being damaged. In animal studies, niacinamide protected against streptozotocin-induced diabetes and inhibited the development of experimental autoimmune diabetes. Niacin administration also prevented the diabetes-inducing effect of alloxan in rabbits and rats. There is evidence that both experimental diabetes and type 1 diabetes in humans are related to a depletion of nicotinamide adenine dinucleotide (NAD) within pancreatic beta cells, resulting in failure of oxidative metabolism and subsequent cell death. As precursors to NAD, niacin and niacinamide are apparently capable of preventing the depletion of NAD in pancreatic beta cells.

Because of its capacity to protect pancreatic beta-cell function, niacinamide has been studied as a possible treatment for newly diagnosed type 1 diabetes, which is characterized by progressive destruction of beta cells. In a double-blind study, 16 type 1 diabetics received either niacinamide (3 g/day) or a placebo, beginning one week after the start of insulin therapy. Insulin was successfully discontinued in 85.7% of the patients taking niacinamide, compared to 55.6% of those taking placebo. Three patients treated with niacinamide for 18 months remained in remission for more than two years. Remissions of such long duration are extremely rare in type 1 diabetes. In another study, 14 children who were at high risk of developing diabetes (as determined by high levels of antibodies against pancreatic islet cells) received either niacinamide (150–300 mg per year of age per day, maximum dose = 3.0 g), while eight children at similar risk served as controls. All eight of the untreated children developed diabetes, compared with only one of the 14 children who received niacinamide. A recent meta-analysis of 10 randomized controlled trials concluded that niacinamide effectively preserves residual pancreatic beta-cell function in children with type 1 diabetes, when treatment is begun at the time of initial diagnosis.

The Promise of Other Vitamins and Minerals

The B-vitamin biotin plays a role in the intracellular metabolism of glucose. Biotin deficiency resulted in impaired glucose tolerance in rats. In another study, administration of biotin (2–4 mg/kg [milligrams per kilograms] of body weight/day) to genetically diabetic mice improved glucose tolerance and lowered insulin resistance.

Biotin has also shown promise in the treatment of diabetes in humans. Seven insulin-dependent diabetics were removed from insulin therapy and treated with biotin (16 mg/day) or a placebo for one week. Fasting blood glucose levels rose significantly in patients given placebo, but decreased significantly in those treated with biotin. In another study, serum biotin levels were significantly lower in 43 patients with non-insulin-dependent diabetes than in healthy controls. Eighteen diabetic patients were given 9 mg/day of biotin for one month, while 10 other patients received a placebo. The mean blood glucose concentration fell by 45% ($p<0.05$) in patients receiving biotin, but did not change in those given placebo.

Biotin has also been used to treat diabetic neuropathy. Three patients with severe diabetic peripheral neuropathy received 10 mg/day of biotin intramuscularly (IM) for six weeks, followed by 10 mg IM three times a week for six weeks, then 5 mg/day orally. The treatment duration ranged from 64 to 130 weeks. Within 4–8 weeks of the start of treatment, painful muscle cramps, paresthesias, and ability to walk improved markedly and restless legs syndrome disappeared.

Serum vitamin B6 levels were below normal in 25% of a series of 518 mostly adult diabetics and in 24% of 63 childhood diabetics. Pyridoxine (vitamin B6) supplementation of diabetic patients improved glucose tolerance in some studies, but was without effect in others. Fourteen women with gestational diabetes were treated with 100 mg/day of pyridoxine for 2 weeks. At the end of the treatment period, 12 of the 14 women no longer had gestational diabetes. The same dosage of vitamin B6 also produced a significant improvement in glucose tolerance in 13 women with late-pregnancy gestational diabetes. Another study failed to confirm the beneficial effect of vitamin B6 on gestational diabetes. However, in that study, the women were hospitalized and confined to a sedentary existence. It is possible that a beneficial effect of vitamin B6 on glucose tolerance was counterbalanced in that study by a lack of activity.

In another study, pyridoxine at a dosage of 50 mg three times per day had no effect on blood glucose but reduced the concentration of glycosylated hemoglobin (HbA1c) by about 6% after six weeks. This finding suggests that vitamin B6 inhibits the glycosylation of proteins and might therefore help prevent diabetic complications.

Vitamin B6 has also been used to treat patients with diabetic neuropathy. Eighteen such patients received 50 mg of pyridoxine three times per day or a placebo for four months. Six (67%) of nine of pyridoxine-treated patients reported significant relief from neuropathic symptoms, compared with 4 (44%) of nine placebo-treated patients. This preliminary report warrants further study. . . .

The importance of vitamin C for blood sugar regulation has been demonstrated in both humans and animals. Guinea pigs fed a vitamin C–deficient diet developed diabetic glucose tolerance curves, glycosuria, and decreased pancreatic insulin content. Diabetic blood sugar curves were also seen in patients with vitamin C deficiency; these values returned to normal after supplementation with vitamin C.

Diabetics are at increased risk of developing vitamin C deficiency. For example, the vitamin C concentrations in plasma, platelets, and white blood cells were significantly lower in diabetics than in healthy controls. Vitamin C deficiency in diabetics may be more pronounced within the cells than in plasma or other body fluids. That is because vitamin C is structurally similar to glucose, and may therefore compete with glucose for transport into cells. In the presence of elevated blood sugar, the uptake of vitamin C into cells appears to be impaired. This reduced entry of vitamin C into certain tissues may result in a kind of "localized scurvy." It is noteworthy that the vascular changes resulting from scurvy resemble those seen in diabetics.

In addition to maintaining the integrity of blood vessels, vitamin C has been shown to inhibit three different biochemical processes that are associated with end-organ damage in diabetics. First, vitamin C functions as an antioxidant. Second, this vitamin inhibits the intracellular accumulation of sorbitol. In one study, supplementation with 2,000 mg/day of vitamin C reduced erythrocyte sorbitol accumulation by 56.1% and 44.5% in healthy individuals and diabetics, respectively. Third, vitamin C significantly reduced the glycosylation of proteins, when given to healthy volunteers at a dose of 1 g [gram]/day. These studies suggest that long-term supplementation with vitamin C may help prevent many of the complications of diabetes.

Injections of vitamin B12 have been used to treat retinopathy in patients with type 1 diabetes. In one study, 15 patients added 100 mcg [micrograms] of vitamin B12 to their daily insulin injection. After one year, all signs of retinopathy had disappeared in seven cases. Similar results were reported by others.

Vitamin B12 has also been used to treat diabetic neuropathy. In one study, 12 patients received 15–30 mcg/day of vitamin B12 by injection for the first 7–14 days, followed by 15–30 mcg, 1–2 times a week. Seven patients had complete or almost complete remission of the neuropathy and three had partial improvement. The response appeared to depend more on the frequency of the injections than on the amount of each individual dose. Other investigators have also found vitamin B12 to be helpful in the treatment of diabetic neuropathy. . . .

The Herbal Treatment of Diabetes

Herbal medicine has been used for many years by different cultures around the world, both for the prevention and treatment of diabetes. It has only been recently that some of these herbal treatments have been studied scientifically.

Fenugreek seed (Trigonella foenumgraecum) is an annual plant of the leguminous family. Fenugreek seeds are commonly used as a condiment in India. Yemenite Jews have traditionally used fenugreek to treat type 2 diabetes. In one study, 10 insulin-dependent diabetics consumed isocaloric diets with or without 100 g/day of debittered, defatted fenugreek-seed powder, each for 10 days in random order. The powder was divided into two equal doses and incorporated into bread. Compared with the control diet, the mean fasting plasma glucose concentration was significantly lower by 28% and glucose tolerance was significantly better during fenugreek treatment. Serum total and LDL-cholesterol levels were also significantly reduced by fenugreek. Similar results were achieved with a lower dose of fenugreek seeds.

The dried sap of the aloe plant is used as a traditional remedy for diabetes in the Arabian peninsula. Administration of one-half teaspoon daily for 4–14 weeks to five patients with non-insulin-dependent diabetes resulted in a mean reduction in serum glucose from 273 to 151 mg/dl [milligrams per deciliter]. Administration of aloes also reduced plasma glucose in alloxan-diabetic mice.

Burdock root has been used traditionally in cases of skin eruptions, gout, and rheumatism. It is commonly used in Japanese cooking. In an uncontrolled study, administration of burdock root in doses of 54–81 g/day reduced insulin requirements in several diabetics. This effect disappeared when the treatment was discontinued; resumption of Burdock root again reduced insulin requirements.

The fruit of Momordica charantia (Bitter Gourd) has been used in traditional herbal medicine for the treatment of rheumatism, gout, dysmenorrhea, jaundice, and disorders of the liver and spleen. Administration of an extract of momordica to mice with alloxan-induced diabetes significantly lowered blood sugar and delayed the onset of retinopathy, nephropathy and cataract. Administration of 230 g/day of momordica for 8–11 weeks to a group of nine diabetic patients, significantly improved the results of oral glucose tolerance tests.

Panax Ginseng, commonly known as Korean ginseng, has a long history of use in Asian countries as a tonic. It is used in China to treat diabetes. At least five constituents of this herb have been shown to exert hypoglycemic effects. In one study, 36 non-insulin-dependent diabetics were randomly assigned to receive ginseng (100 or 200 mg per day) or a placebo for eight weeks (the type of ginseng was not specified). Compared with placebo, treatment with ginseng lowered blood sugar levels and improved mood and psychological performance. The 200-mg dose of ginseng was more effective than the lower dose.

CHAPTER 4

LIVING WITH DIABETES

THE SECRETS OF MY SUCCESS: A DIABETIC TAKES CONTROL

Richard K. Daly, as told to Peggy Morgan

Richard K. Daly got a wake-up call in 1996 when he was diagnosed with diabetes. In the following selection, Daly tells Peggy Morgan, a staff writer for *Prevention* magazine, how he took control of his diabetes by altering his lifestyle. Before he was diagnosed, Daly drank sugary cola drinks and ate refined foods such as Twinkies and potato chips. After his stay in the hospital, however, Daly changed his diet and began a walking program. As a result, Morgan reports, he was able to discontinue all his diabetes management drugs. Daly says he feels like a new person. *Prevention* is a popular health, nutrition, and fitness magazine.

Back in the early 1980s—long before it was popular in my neck of the Michigan woods—I started a walking program. Actually, it was a *yo-yo* walking program: winters in Port Huron are so severe that my exercise disappeared from late fall to late spring. Treadmills and club memberships were too expensive and, back then, we didn't have indoor malls to walk in. I basically hibernated through the winters. My only physical activity was reaching for Twinkies, cakes, and pies.

When spring rolled around, I'd start walking again. Every walking season, I'd lose about 18 pounds. And every winter, I'd gain almost 30. You don't need a math degree to figure out what was happening. But *I* failed to make the calculations.

Over the years I back-and-forthed my weight up to 244 pounds. At that point, it took me longer to finish a typical walk, and I was tired most of the time. I also had an almost unquenchable thirst. One night in April 1996, I looked down at the floor beside my easy chair and counted eight cola cans that I'd emptied in less than an hour.

A Wake-Up Call

The next thing I knew I was in the hospital, diagnosed with diabetes. For five days, I was there getting insulin to bring down my sky-high blood sugar and learning how to give myself shots of insulin. However, the diabetes education classes, which drove home the impor-

From "I Whipped Diabetes and Got Off All Meds! My Doctor's Amazed," by Richard K. Daly, as told to Peggy Morgan, *Prevention*, March 1998. Copyright © 1998 by Rodale, Inc. Reprinted with permission.

tance of a healthy diet, exercising, checking product labels, and testing my blood sugar levels, inspired me to take control.

My first morning home from the hospital, I started a *real* walking program. Every day, rain or snow, I walked at least 35 minutes. When the weather was bad, I walked in the mall or on the treadmill I bought. (I now considered it a *necessary* expense!) I started walking the 2 miles to and from work too.

My hospitalization also convinced me to start eating right. Instead of highly refined cakes and cookies, I began reading labels and buying unrefined foods such as fruits, vegetables, whole grain breads, and cereals. I also started eating oatmeal and bran cereal—with skim milk and raspberries or blueberries for more flavor.

I'd eat three meals a day. Then, about 2 or 3 hours after a meal, I'd have a snack—fruit, cottage cheese, a bagel, or carrots instead of chips. If I got an urge for something sweet, I'd have a piece of fruit instead of the usual Twinkie.

At restaurants, I'd stick with baked or broiled fish. Every once in a while, I'd indulge. One day at work I'd have a hot pork sandwich, potatoes, and peas—the works. But then I'd eat lighter at dinner—a piece of turkey breast and a salad. I really didn't feel like I was dieting. The one thing I did give up, though, were my Friday night all-you-can-eat fish fries. They no longer appealed to my taste buds, nor to the new, health-conscious me.

Fitting Rewards

A month after I got home from the hospital, I was off insulin and only on a small dose of medication. Within two months, I was off all drugs. My body fat started coming off even faster. And some women friends began to look at me with more interest.

That first summer, I realized that I was losing a little *too* much weight, probably because the nice weather was allowing me to exercise even more. So I increased my intake, being careful that those additional calories came from healthy foods. When people look at my plate, they're often surprised at how much I can eat and still keep my weight where it should be.

About that time I also started working out with dumbbells three times a week.

A year after I left the hospital, my weight was down to 170 pounds—a 74-pound loss! I've maintained it ever since. My waist is 10 inches smaller, and I'm fit, lean, and muscular. My blood sugar is below 100 (milligrams per deciliter of blood) from a high in the hospital of 290. My doctor still shakes his head in amazement at what I've accomplished.

The "new me" sleeps better and has plenty of energy. At 61, I feel better than I've ever felt.

TAKING THE OFFENSIVE AGAINST TYPE 1 DIABETES

Kerry Pianoforte

Cincinnati Bengals offensive lineman Jay Leeuwenburg was diagnosed with Type 1 diabetes at the age of twelve, writes Kerry Pianoforte in the following selection. In order to prevent Leeuwenburg from feeling different from other children, the author reports, his family adopted a team approach to dealing with his diabetes. Because Leeuwenburg wanted to remain active in sports, he and his family educated his coaches and teammates to eliminate their fears. Leeuwenburg is able to pursue a career in football because he rigorously monitors his blood sugar and adjusts his insulin to match his eating and activity schedule, says Pianoforte. According to the author, Leeuwenburg shares this offensive strategy when he speaks to children, and using his experience as an example, Leeuwenburg encourages children to take control of their diabetes and do whatever they choose to do in life. Pianoforte is a staff writer for *The Exceptional Parent,* a magazine that provides information and support for parents and families of children with disabilities.

In football, offensive linemen form the "brick wall" that protects the quarterback from the onslaught of the opposing team's defense. On the playing field, Jay Leeuwenburg, the 6'3", 290 lb. offensive lineman for the Cincinnati Bengals, stands his ground. Off the field, Jay Leeuwenburg does not let anything, especially his diabetes, stand in the way of his dreams. Jay was diagnosed at the age of 12 with Type 1, or "juvenile," diabetes. This lifelong condition, which affects more than one million Americans, can occur at any age, but is most commonly diagnosed in childhood. In Type 1 diabetes, the pancreas produces little or no life-sustaining insulin. People with this condition must take several insulin injections a day for the rest of their lives. Before being diagnosed with juvenile diabetes, Jay had some of the classic symptoms such as an unquenchable thirst, frequent urination, and lethargy. The diagnosis was a shock for Jay and his family because

From "The Best Offense Is a Good Defense," by Kerry Pianoforte, *The Exceptional Parent,* March 2000. Copyright © 2000 by Psy-Ed Corporation. Reprinted with permission.

there was no family history of the disease. He felt relief, however, upon receiving a diagnosis and proper treatment. He recalls, "I think I felt so bad from having been undiagnosed that as soon as I got my first shot of insulin I felt so much better."

A Team Effort

Jay credits his parent's approach to his illness with helping him enjoy a happy childhood. "They did a great job of making ours a 'diabetic' family." Jay explains that as a family they all kept to the carefully balanced diet that he required to help keep his disease under control. "I have an older brother and never did I feel that because I have diabetes I missed out on something." Jay feels that this "team" approach to diabetes is important because, "children hate to feel different, they hate to feel alienated, and it is important to make them feel like they are still as normal as possible. People have to realize, particularly as a child, if you are going to a birthday party you're going to have cake and ice cream because it is important for you to fit in. You have to compensate by having less pizza, and you may have to take more insulin." This team approach is something Jay still practices at his home with wife Ingher and their two young daughters. "If I know that I'm going out and having dessert, I'll take some more insulin. As long as you have a little forethought and you actually think about what you're doing rather than doing whatever you want, you can reach a balance. I don't think it's dependent on whether you're diabetic or not, I think it's fairly good practice for everyone."

Throughout his life, Jay has defied the odds with his "can do" attitude. Jay would not allow diabetes to slow him down. "I always knew that I wanted to be active. Sports was a priority in my life, even as a child." Jay stresses that parents should encourage their children to pursue any activity, regardless of a disability. The NFL lineman believes that parents can help by eliminating any fear of the unknown on the part of others. "The key to a successful experience, whether it be in sports or in the marching band, is education. Educate the coach or leader on the signs of the illness and then explain how it is treated. This avoids any fear of the unknown." Jay and his parents took this up-front approach and explained his illness to his coaches and teammates from the beginning. Even now, in the NFL, he is always willing to answer questions concerning diabetes.

After coming to terms with diabetes and understanding its treatment, Jay played football in high school, where he was a starting member of the football team. His football career continued at the University of Colorado, where he was selected as one of only four athletes in the university's athletic history to be nominated as a unanimous All American. Jay started his NFL career first with the Chicago Bears, followed by the Indianapolis Colts, and he is now with the Cincinnati Bengals.

Setting an Example

Jay is actively involved in the Juvenile Diabetes Foundation. He spends much of his free time speaking to children about the importance of taking care of oneself when you have this disease. Jay advises that children should not feel limited because of their disease, and parents should not fear letting their children try new things. Jays feels that "any individual who has diabetes can do whatever he or she wants, but they have to take some important steps. It's different for every individual with diabetes, but there are some universals like checking your sugars, being on a diet, getting exercise, and taking your insulin."

Jay is able to maintain a physically rigorous schedule by constantly monitoring his blood sugar. Using his blood glucose monitor, he checks his sugar eight to ten times a day on a non-game day and even more frequently on a game day. This allows Jay to have tighter control over his disease by adjusting his insulin according to his blood sugar for that day. He also suggests that individuals develop a system tailored to their needs by talking to their doctor or diabetes educator.

One of the reasons that Jay Leeuwenburg has dedicated himself to being a role model for children is because he did not know of any people who had diabetes that he could look up to when he was a child. He hopes that children will see the example that he sets and realize that people with diabetes can do anything they set their minds to. Jay cannot stress enough how important it is to take insulin shots. "The way I think of it now is that insulin is just life support until they find a cure."

Jay has hope that someday in the near future there will be a cure for this disease. With his work with the Juvenile Diabetes Foundation he hopes to raise awareness and educate young people on maintaining their health. Jay advises that people stay informed about the latest advances in diabetes research. "I like to stick with what works, but I found out there are better ways that I can be monitoring and living my life with diabetes. There's new technology, new insulins, and meters."

Jay has no plans of slowing down. Right now he is busy balancing the demands of family life, being an NFL player, and his obligations as a spokesperson for the Juvenile Diabetes Foundation. Jay wants parents and children alike to understand that diabetes does not have to limit you. Parents need to educate themselves to better understand the disease. Children need to know that with proper healthcare, they can lead active, healthy lives. As Jay would say "You need to control your diabetes, not let your diabetes control you." This sound, offensive strategy will control any defense, and any disability.

A Curse of Diabetes Becomes a Blessing

Tom Thompkins

When Tom Thompkins first learned that he had type 2 diabetes, he saw the disease as a death sentence. However, with the support of his family, Thompkins took control of his diabetes, watching his diet and even visualizing high-carbohydrate foods as poison. As a result, Thompkins brought down his blood sugar and began to lose weight. After implementing an exercise program, Thompkins eventually lost a total of sixty-two pounds. Thompkins concluded that the "curse" of diabetes forced him to take control of his life and health, which proved, in fact, to be a blessing. Tom Thompkins is a writer from Woodland Hills, California, who writes on medical issues for publications such as *Vibrant Life*, a magazine that promotes healthful living.

As a patient I was stunned. As a medical professional I found it simply the final confirmation of the suspicions I had secretly carried for the past several months. The symptoms had become far too obvious for me to ignore any longer—an all-consuming thirst, frequent urination, constant exhaustion, and steady weight gain—so I finally called a trusted friend and told her my suspicions.

Dr. Lois Jovanovic, director of Sansum Clinic in Santa Barbara, California, and an internationally recognized diabetes expert, had a few choice words for me for not calling her sooner, and then ordered me to her office immediately. The blood tests she performed when I walked in the door confirmed what we both already knew. I had the same disease that had caused my father's slow, miserable death; and I thus became a statistic, adding my name to the long list of 16 million diagnosed and undiagnosed diabetics in the United States.

A Bleak Future

I listened to Dr. Jovanovic in stunned silence, accepting the diagnosis with the same sense of resignation that a person accepts a death sentence being handed down by a judge. I saw my father when he was barely 10 years older than my present age, suffering those long-term complications I now saw in my future—blindness, kidney failure, multiple circulatory complications, and ultimately, heart disease. We found him with his nitroglycerin tablets spilled on the floor beside his bed.

She explained that Type II diabetes—formerly known as adult-onset or non-insulin-dependent diabetes mellitus—is by far the most common form of diabetes, affecting 85 to 90 percent of all diabetics. It is sometimes referred to as "insulin-resistant diabetes," because while the body manufactures adequate amounts of insulin, Type II diabetics are unable to utilize the insulin that is produced (contrasted to Type I diabetes, in which the pancreas fails to manufacture insulin in sufficient amounts). Since cells require insulin in order to break down glucose into energy, high levels of glucose are trapped uselessly in the bloodstream, explaining why uncontrolled or undiagnosed diabetics suffer from chronic exhaustion. Its insidious onset often masks the disease for many years, postponing the diagnosis until one of the long-term complications appears. In a sense, then, I was "lucky" to have discovered it as early as I did.

On the way home I called my wife on my cell phone, and barely got the words out before I choked on them. I was not prepared to face my own mortality with such vivid memories clouding my vision. In the calm supportive voice I have grown to love over the years she said, "Don't worry. We'll handle this together." I knew she meant it.

Taking Control

I withdrew from social life and turned inward. My medications, my diet, and the full-time task of feeling sorry for myself became the entire focus of my existence. At 276 pounds and with a blood sugar of 337 (normal range is 80–120), I knew I had a long uncomfortable road ahead of me. But I intended to force it upon no one outside my own family. I have always been a very private person, and this became my own personal battle.

A week later my fingertips had become reluctant pincushions and my medicine cabinet was, for the first time in my life, filled with prescription medicines and blood-testing paraphernalia. My family was coping with my dietary restrictions with gentle, yet firm, commitment. Their constant encouragement buoyed my flagging spirits, and the game of reading food labels became an enjoyable part of our trips to the grocery store. Even my teenage son got into the spirit of things, checking my meals to make sure I wasn't cheating.

I began attaching the mental label of "poison" to high-carbohydrate foods, trying to give myself an image that would make it easier to avoid the foods that would drive my blood sugar dangerously high again. Believe me, seeing the skull and crossbones wavering in the ether mist over a piece of my wife's steaming hot pecan pie was truly a nightmarish experience.

A New Attitude

It didn't take long before my efforts began yielding noticeable results. My blood sugar came under control in surprisingly short order. At my one-month follow-up visit I had lost 15 pounds, and my blood sugar was actually a bit low—low enough, in fact, that Dr. Jovanovic cut my medications in half. The sweet smell of success was beginning to replace the loss of that pecan pie. Another month, and I had dropped a total of 25 pounds. I reached a plateau another month later at 235 pounds, at which point my clothes were literally beginning to fall off me. I finally felt that I could begin exercising in earnest, and now, eight months after being diagnosed, I weigh 214 pounds. *That's 62 pounds less than where I started!*

I run two miles each morning; my blood sugar recently was 96, and I have energy again. In short, I feel like a new person. My attitude toward life and my disease is greatly different from what it was that first morning when Dr. Jovanovic confronted me with what I perceived as a "death sentence." I am fast approaching the point at which medication may no longer be necessary, and Dr. Jovanovic has begun referring to me as her "diabetes poster child."

For me, the curse of being given the label of "diabetic" has turned into the blessing of a lifetime. It forced me to get control of my life and my health. I accept full responsibility for the management of both, and pursue them with a degree of vigor and enthusiasm I thought had long since left me. Lois Jovanovic told me that I would one day be thankful for my diabetes, and I could not for the life of me understand what she meant. Now I do. So I say, "Thank You, God, for giving me diabetes. And thank You for making my life worth living again."

LEARNING THE IMPORTANCE OF TALKING ABOUT DIABETES

Christen Opsal

While a student at the University of Wisconsin, in Madison, Christen Opsal discovered she had diabetes. Although she was frightened, she was surprised to discover how many people in her college community were willing to help and support her. In the following selection, Opsal reveals how her experience taught her the value of a support community and how talking to others about her struggle with diabetes helped her learn to cope. According to Opsal, by talking about her experiences she was able to help others who suffered from diseases that can be physically, mentally, and emotionally frustrating. Opsal was a student of history and religious studies at the time this selection was written.

Ira Sleeps Over, a delightful children's book by Bernard Waber, tells the story of Ira, a little boy who wants to bring his teddy bear with him when he goes to sleep over at his friend Reggie's house. His parents think that this is a good idea. "Of course you should bring your teddy bear," they say. But his older sister doesn't agree. "Reggie will laugh," she says. Ira believes his sister and leaves his teddy bear at home when he goes to Reggie's. That night, as the boys get ready for bed, Reggie introduces Ira to his own teddy bear. Ira immediately excuses himself and rushes home (in his pajamas!) to bring his teddy bear to join the slumber party.

Like Ira, I have often been afraid that others might not accept things that are important to me. I was recently diagnosed with diabetes, a condition that made me feel vulnerable and unsure of myself. At the same time, however, I found myself unable to separate my diabetes from Me, and therefore I felt compelled to share what had happened to me with people I care about. The following is the story of that sharing, sharing that taught me, as it did Ira, that other people have vulnerabilities very like my own.

I thought I had a cold I couldn't get rid of. I spent 2 weeks sneezing and sniffling, only to spend still another week sleeping and downing fluids. I was lethargic and skipped class to nap. One day, I was awake for a total of only 5 hours. By then, I knew I had more than a cold, but I could not stay awake long enough to discern what.

Then came the morning I woke up and couldn't see very well. Even with my glasses on, the world was fuzzy around the edges. That was Friday. On Saturday, my sight still had not returned. Alone in my dorm room that afternoon, I had a hunch. I went to my computer and searched the web for "diabetes." Reading the symptoms on the American Diabetes Association's (ADA) web site was eerie. I had them all: excessive thirst and urination, unexplained weight loss, and weakness, in addition to fatigue and blurred vision. Fear came first, settling in my chest and knotting my throat. A sense of relieved hope followed—not enough to overwhelm the fear, but enough to keep me going until I knew for sure.

Soon, my two roommates came home. I had resolved not to worry about it, so I didn't share my hypothesis with them until another friend showed up later that night to invite me to go swing dancing. Responding that I wouldn't be able to see my dance partner, I sobbed, "I think I have diabetes" and spilled the whole story.

Then my friend remembered that one of my dorm mates had recently been diagnosed with diabetes. She phoned him, and soon he and his glucometer were on their way. By this time, thanks to an open door, our small dorm room was slowly filling with curious neighbors. So when Adam arrived, I was reluctantly and shakily sharing what was going on and why. My concerned floor mates watched as he pricked my finger and soon welcomed me to the "Diabetes Club." My blood glucose was 340, some 200 points above the normal range.

Four of us went to a local emergency room, where I saw a doctor who gave me little physical relief but much emotional comfort. His assessment of my condition was only a confirmation that something was wrong and that I needed to see someone about it on Monday. But I knew that somehow my plight mattered to him when he revealed that his own college-age daughter had recently been diagnosed with diabetes. He even called a few days later to see how I was doing.

By Monday morning, my mom was on her way to Madison, Wisconsin, from Minneapolis, Minnesota, and I had an appointment to be seen at our campus health service. That one appointment turned into a full day of testing and education. Two days later, the diagnosis—type 1 diabetes—was confirmed. Having been treated with insulin since Monday, my sight was back, my sugar was down, and I was feeling nearly normal.

My "diabetes week" ended with a mass e-mail I sent to friends and colleagues a few days later. In it, I told them of the diagnosis, answered some already-common questions, and asked for their support and understanding. Some replied, offering words of encouragement. Others gave me cards, hugs, flowers, diabetic cookbooks, and, most important, opportunities to talk about my experience—how it felt to be diagnosed with a chronic medical condition and what it meant for me.

But my struggle with diabetes won't end until I do. It's been humbling and a bit scary for me to admit that I have a life-endangering medical condition. I feel as though it means I'm a less-than-perfect person, and by admitting my obstacles to a "normal" life, I risk sounding whiny or hypochondriac. But having been diagnosed with diabetes, and most important, sharing that diagnosis with people around me, has instead taught me that my life and good health matter to others.

Even better, though, is that sharing my diabetes experience freed others to share their own physical, mental, and emotional struggles with me. I recently talked with Gary, a University of Wisconsin staff member who suffers from rheumatoid arthritis, about living with a chronic physical condition: who you need to tell, what personal limitations you have to accept. Stacy, another student, aired her struggles with manic depressive disorder. Sarah, a close friend being treated for depression during the same time I was learning to deal with diabetes, shared the frustration of a condition that affects physical, mental, and emotional well-being all at once.

Adam and I continue to swap diabetes resources, advice, and stories. And of course, everybody has a relative with diabetes who they have to tell me about. But I value the firsthand experience of Gary, Stacy, Sarah, and Adam more.

Discovering a Support Community

As you can see, throughout my diabetes story thus far, I have been surrounded by people who communicated their support and empathy in many different ways. In retrospect, I feel as though I have learned more about the give and take of community in those harrowing days than in years of "belonging" to clubs and organizations. Nothing obliged my neighbors to huddle around me as Adam pricked my finger; genuine, spontaneous human concern brought them in. The doctor from the emergency room didn't have to check up on me, but he did, perhaps because he had seen his own daughter's fear on my face that night. My friends listened, whereas other people would stammer, "Diabetes? Oh, I'm sorry," and change the subject.

My diabetes experience has also taught me that we can cultivate community through consciously sharing our lives and stories with each other. Although everyone may not have a strong network of friends and family with whom they feel comfortable sharing significant things, I feel that we keep things from others—friends, family, even professionals—at our own peril. Not being able to share, out of fear or pride or both, is itself a woe. In the December 7, 1998, issue actor Michael J. Fox, who recently made public his ongoing struggle

with Parkinson's disease, told *People* magazine about what it meant
for him to share the condition with those around him:

> It's not that I had a deep, dark secret. It was just my thing to
> deal with. But this box I had put everything into kind of
> expanded to a point where it's difficult to lug around. What's
> inside the box isn't inhibiting me. It's the box itself. I think I
> can help people by talking. I want to help myself and my
> family.

In his new book, *Love and Survival,* Dr. Dean Ornish recounts several
studies of heart disease and cancer patients. Those who attended support group meetings as part of their treatment fared better in the long
run. Those who didn't share their sufferings were more likely to lead
shorter, less healthy lives. Why? Because sharing connects us with other
people. Reservation multiplies our woes; sharing diminishes them.

Sharing may be difficult to initiate. In fact, I believe the difficulty
of talking about certain things is often directly proportionate to the
importance of talking about them. The more important talking about
something is, the more difficult it will be. Remember that big conversations come only after the trust built in small conversations.

With Ornish and Fox, I have learned that our health relies on the
sharing act of meaningful communication—the exchange of words,
ideas, and feelings. I agree that sharing, whether teddy bears or type 1
diabetes, lessens woes, builds bonds, helps us feel as though we matter
to others, and therefore makes us more inclined to live fully.

Breaking the Cycle of Diabetes

Marie McCarren

Marie McCarren is associate editor of *Diabetes Forecast*, a publication of the American Diabetes Association (ADA). In the following selection, she relates the experience of Letitia Thomas who in 1994 concluded that she and her children were at risk for diabetes and decided to do what she could to prevent the onset of the disease. Thomas discovered that she exhibited many of the risk factors that contribute to the onset of diabetes: she was African American, overweight, had a family history of diabetes, and had developed gestational diabetes while pregnant with both her children. Since Thomas had no control over her ethnicity and family history, the author reports, she took control of what she could—her family's lifestyle and eating habits. Her family was reluctant at first, particularly her husband and her mother, both of whom already had diabetes, but when they realized diet and exercise could alleviate the complications of diabetes, they too began to accept Thomas's suggestions. McCarren also describes research by the National Institute of Diabetes and Digestive and Kidney Diseases (NIDDK). In 1996, the institute began the Diabetes Prevention Program (DPP), a study to test the success of diet, exercise, and drug therapy in preventing diabetes for those at risk. Subsequent to the publication of this article, the researchers completed the study and concluded that a low-fat diet and exercise can reduce the risk of getting type 2 diabetes by 58 percent.

You want to talk "at risk," talk to Letitia Thomas. Two years ago, she took stock of all the things that put her at risk for developing type 2 diabetes.

Adding Up the Risk Factors

First, her family history. Her maternal grandmother, now dead, had diabetes. Her mother, Delma Johnson, 60, was diagnosed with diabetes at age 42. "I've been overweight all my life," says Johnson, "so I knew I wouldn't escape it. I just didn't know it would be that quick."

Thomas' brother was diagnosed at age 22.

Letitia Thomas knew type 2 diabetes runs in families, so she understood that she was at risk for diabetes herself. There was another factor working against her: her own history. Thomas has two sons, Antione, 12, and Antonio, 7. During both pregnancies, Thomas developed mild gestational diabetes. According to some studies, 40 percent of women with a history of gestational diabetes develop type 2 diabetes within 20 years.

Thomas added another mark because of her race. African Americans, as well as Hispanics and Native Americans, are at higher risk for type 2 diabetes than non-Hispanic whites.

Finally, Thomas added a mark for her weight. "All along, from age 18, I tried to lose weight. But I didn't have my mind on it." Two years ago, at age 28, the 5'3" Thomas weighed 234 pounds. Obesity, Thomas knew, raised her risk of type 2 diabetes.

Thomas figured her diabetes was just around the corner, waiting for her. So she hit the brakes and turned the other way.

"All of a sudden, I thought, If I don't take control of this now, I'll get to where I can't," she says.

Changing the Family's Eating Habits

Thomas took hold of the one risk factor she could control. "One morning I woke up and said, I'm going on a diet."

She switched to eating healthier, low-fat food and exercised more. "I've always liked walking," she says. "But when I was eating what I wanted to, walking didn't help my weight." She kept up with the walking, and added workouts on a Cardio-Glide, a type of home exercise equipment. Thomas lost 45 pounds in a year and is working on losing 25 more.

At first, she says, her family wasn't too keen on the change in their meals. Her mother, who lives with the Thomases, would simply say, "No, thank you" to the meals Thomas prepared, and go into the kitchen and fry some chicken or fish. Thomas' husband, James, called the new meals "rabbit food."

But then, slowly, James Thomas came to his wife's way of thinking. Two years ago, at age 29, he was told by his doctor that he had diabetes. At first, he refused to believe it. "I was like: He doesn't know what he's talking about," says James Thomas.

"The doctor said we would try to control it through my diet. He told me he was sending me to a dietitian. But I was being hard-headed and didn't see the dietitian."

Her husband's diabetes made Letitia Thomas even more determined to change her family's eating habits. Not for her husband's sake, not for her own sake, but for her sons'.

"They have a double dose of risk—from my side of the family and from their father's" she says. "I thought, If I don't make changes now, they'll grow up with bad habits." She decided three generations of diabetes were enough, and she redoubled her efforts to get her family on the right track.

"My wife would get on my back to eat right," James Thomas recalls, "and I'd say, 'I'm doing all right, I'm doing it.' But I wasn't doing it."

Thomas found himself getting up in the middle of the night to urinate, and he was tired all the time. "As time went on, I could see what the doctor was talking about. I started trying to follow the doctor's directions."

Making an About-Face

By that time, James Thomas' blood glucose was high enough that his doctor prescribed diabetes pills. But Thomas knew he needed to do more.

"My father is diabetic, and he never took care of himself," he says. "He just took his needle, and he thought he was invincible. One time his sugar went up to 800, and he went into a coma. He's had heart surgery."

So, like his wife had done, James Thomas made a dietary about-face. "I started living the way I'm supposed to," he says.

When he was first diagnosed, Thomas was working at a fast-food restaurant. A typical breakfast was two ham-egg-cheese croissants, hash browns, and three orange juices. For lunch, he'd grab the biggest hamburger on the menu. For dinner: a triple hamburger with cheese. And he drank regular sodas like other people drink water.

"I changed my diet myself," says Thomas, who now sells life insurance. "I stopped eating sugar, period. I cut down on eating a loaf of bread a day, quit eating a lot of fried foods, and the weight fell right off."

He's gone from 296 pounds to 252, helped in part by his workouts on the Cardio-Glide.

"My weight has been steady for the past six months," he says. "What we're working on now is me lowering my calorie intake. I figure I can lose another 20 or 25 pounds."

To that end, he has seen a dietitian twice, with another visit scheduled.

"I'm fully aware of my diet now," he says. "Instead of eating candy as a snack, I'll eat pretzels. Some of the things that my wife eats, I learned to like: granola bars, baked chicken. I don't eat fried chicken at all. It still smells the same, and I know that the taste of fried chicken is good, but it just doesn't attract me.

"I still don't do all the things that my wife wants me to. I'm not supposed to eat a lot of rolls, but I have a soft spot in my heart for hot rolls. So last time we went out, I ate four instead of a half dozen. I was still hungry, so I ate some rabbit food—a salad.

"It's not that my wife nags, she really cares what I do. I try to live the way she wants me to. It's better. I can see the difference. I don't run to the bathroom all through the night and feel tired during the day. Physically, I feel a lot better, a lot stronger.

"I really want to be around for my kids, and I want to live a longer life for my wife, so we can enjoy life. In 10 years, our kids will be old enough to be on their own, and we'll still be young."

Now that Letitia Thomas has her husband's support, she is realizing her goal of a healthier family. Her elder son, Antione, recently realized he was getting too heavy and has started to count calories and eat lower-fat food.

The Type 2 Prevention Program

Letitia Thomas is betting that healthy eating, exercise, and weight loss will prevent her and her sons from getting type 2 diabetes. She's in good company. Researchers at the National Institute of Diabetes and Digestive and Kidney Diseases (NIDDK), part of the National Institutes of Health, agree—and they're out to prove it.

In June 1996, NIDDK launched the Diabetes Prevention Program (DPP). Over the next four years, at 25 medical centers across the country, 4,000 people at high risk will try to avoid developing diabetes.

Thomas works at Johns Hopkins School of Medicine, in Baltimore, one of the 25 centers. Once the DPP starts, she'll be doing data entry for the study. She might end up entering data on her sisters, whom she is encouraging to get screened for the study. She hasn't had much luck yet—"they're hard-headed"—but recruitment for the study will continue for four years, and Thomas will keep working on her sisters. "Three of them are short and overweight," she says. "I try to encourage them to join by reminding them that there's a weight-loss program in the study."

Thomas' sisters certainly have plenty of risk factors for diabetes, but the NIDDK researchers are taking only those people whose blood tests show that they are at very high risk of developing diabetes.

Let's say, for example, that Letitia Thomas convinces one of her sisters to be screened. One day, that sister will skip breakfast and have blood drawn. If her glucose level is high, that may mean she already has diabetes.

That's one advantage to being screened. It's estimated that, on average, people have type 2 diabetes for six years before they are diagnosed. Some people already have complications when they are diagnosed. Although no one likes to hear that they have diabetes, it's best to know and have it treated as soon as possible.

If the fasting blood glucose level is just moderately high, Thomas' sister will be given a sugary drink. Two hours later, her blood will be drawn again. If her blood glucose level is high then, it means that her body did not handle the sugar as quickly as it should have. That's called impaired glucose tolerance (IGT).

Eleven percent of the adults in the United States have impaired glucose tolerance. Out of every 100 people with IGT whose fasting blood glucose level is 100 to 139 milligrams per deciliter (mg/dl), about 7 of them will develop diabetes each year. That's each year—not 7 total. The Diabetes Prevention Program will test whether diet, exercise, weight loss, or pills will lower the number of people with IGT who go on to diabetes.

The Study

About 200,000 people age 25 and older will be screened for the study, until researchers have the 4,000 people with IGT that they need. More than half will be from ethnic groups at high risk for developing diabetes: African Americans, Hispanic Americans, American Indians, Asian Americans, and Pacific Islanders. About 20 percent of the volunteers will be age 65 or older. As subjects are identified, they'll be randomly assigned to one of four groups, assigned a case manager, and then tracked for three to six years (depending on when they joined).

One fourth of the volunteers will be placed in the Intensive Lifestyle group. These people will have Lifestyle Coaches, who will help them eat healthy diets designed to help them lose—and keep off—7 percent of their weight. The weight loss goal will be 1 to 2 pounds per week, with the final weight goal to be achieved after 24 weeks.

Exercise will be encouraged. By five weeks into the study, participants will be doing two and a half hours of moderate physical activity (such as brisk walking) a week. At least twice a week, each study center will sponsor supervised activities, perhaps at the local YMCA, mall, or park.

For the first six months, each participant will see his or her Lifestyle Coach every week or two, and then at least every other month for the rest of the study.

But the NIDDK isn't testing only weight loss. A second group of volunteers will get standard (but not intensive) guidance about following a healthy diet and exercising more often. They'll also take metformin once a day. Metformin is a medication used to treat type 2 diabetes. Several studies suggest it may prevent diabetes.

A third group of volunteers will take troglitazone. This drug has recently been approved in Japan to treat diabetes and is being studied in the United States. Studies indicate it may help people avoid diabetes.

A fourth group, the control group, will get standard advice on diet and exercise, and will not take any study medication. . . .

If you have type 2 diabetes, your blood relatives are at risk. You probably know other people who are at risk. Your daughter-in-law had gestational diabetes? She's at risk.

That tenor you sing next to in choir who's 30 pounds overweight and who confided to you that he's worried about diabetes because his father had it? He's at risk.

Knowing what you know now, if you could have prevented your diabetes, you probably would have. Even a delay of diabetes would have helped your body. Every year of delay is one less year of the higher-than-normal blood glucose levels that are linked to complications.

You've got the benefit of hindsight. Your friends and relatives don't. Maybe you could lend them some of yours and encourage those who are at risk for developing type 2 diabetes to get tested for IGT.

Most of the time, encouraging other people to get healthier is a thankless job. But think of the benefits to you.

Say your daughter-in-law had gestational diabetes during her last pregnancy. After receiving information from you, she gets tested and finds out she's got impaired glucose tolerance. She changes how she cooks for her family. That helps her. It also helps her husband, who is at risk for diabetes because he's related to you. . . .

You don't think it'll work? Consider the change in Letitia Thomas' family. Even her mother is changing her ways. "I used to fry everything I ate," says Delma Johnson. "Bacon, sausage, chicken—whatever meat I had, I used to fry it, mostly every day.

"Now I eat fried chicken maybe once a week, or every other week. I changed because it was better for me, and I changed because my daughter kept after me."

Johnson also went to see a dietitian last year, and she intends to improve her diet even more, with the help of her daughter.

"I'm going to eat what she cooks—but I won't be eating it so gladly," she says, laughing. But then she allows, "It tastes OK. She seasons pretty well. I'm getting to learn to like it.

"I feel better, and I see it's helping my diabetes. I'm going to stay with the way she cooks."

James Thomas says, "We're all looking a little more healthy, all eating healthier foods. Rabbit food looks better and better."

Taking a Chance on Islet Transplantation

Adam Marcus

The transplanting of insulin-producing islet cells into the pancreases of type 1 diabetics is considered by some researchers to be the best treatment available for those who must have daily insulin shots. However, in the following selection, Adam Marcus reports that the procedure has met with mixed success. Marcus relates the story of one patient, for example, who has not needed insulin shots for over two years and has had little reaction to the immune-suppressing drugs necessary to keep the body from rejecting the transplanted cells. The author reveals the stories of other patients, however, whose bodies rejected the cells or who experience severe reactions to the immune-suppressing drugs. Despite these problems, says Marcus, most patients believe the transplants were worth the risk. Marcus is a senior staff writer for *HealthScout News*, a news service that specializes in health issues.

In June 2000, Canadian researchers announced a landmark treatment for Type 1 diabetes that freed a small group of patients from daily insulin shots for as long as a year.

The treatment, a transplant of insulin-producing islet cells from the pancreas and a regimen of drugs for the immune system, was so successful that it was expanded from seven patients to 15. Three more are just getting started.

But a year later, the success is somewhat tempered. Though the doctors still believe the needle-free treatment is better than anything that came before it, five of those 15 patients are back on the daily shots typical of the disease.

"We of course would have liked 100 percent success. But this is better than any other prior" attempt at transplanting islet cells, says Dr. Edmond Ryan, medical director of the islet cell transplant program, now known as the Edmonton Protocol.

For nearly 40 years, Robert Teskey was a slave to needles. Diagnosed with diabetes as a child, Teskey needed daily shots of the hormone insulin to keep his blood sugar in balance.

All that changed in 1999, when the Edmonton lawyer, now 54, enrolled in a University of Alberta study to give him insulin-producing islet cells harvested from dead people. Type 1 diabetics like Teskey destroy their own islet cells through a mutiny of their immune system, and gradually lose the ability to generate the hormone, which helps muscles convert glucose into energy.

Before the islet cell grafts, Teskey's blood sugar levels fluctuated wildly, dropping to 2 on the Canadian glucose scale and spiking to 30 in a single day. "The high and low swings really do dramatically sap your energy and can ruin a day. And you have those swings most days," Teskey says. Since the procedure, Teskey says his blood glucose hovers in a range between 5 and 7—healthy and normal.

And the blackouts and weakness? "That doesn't happen at all any more," he says.

Then there's Don Cammidge. Cammidge, of Edmonton, is one of the patients for whom the transplant procedure has been bittersweet. One of the first to get the grafts in December 1999, the 36-year-old furniture store owner is now on his third set of islet cells, having lost most of the first two to viral infections.

"I have to take a little bit of insulin still at night, but the situation's better than it used to be. It's a lot better."

The Alberta researchers have completed the grafts in 15 patients and have three more in the early stages of the procedure. Of that group, 10—including Teskey—no longer need daily insulin but five others have backslid, says Ryan.

The scientists are now investigating why the grafts have worked better in some patients than in others, analyzing blood samples and other characteristics for clues.

Islets normally reside in the pancreas, but the transplanted cells, some 800,000 in all, are injected into the liver. Some are almost certainly dying off, but how many and why isn't clear, says Ryan, who presented a roundup of the program's progress and the early findings at a meeting of diabetes researchers in June 2001.

Islet grafts "can help a small number of patients, but as far as really helping the diabetes problem, it will really be unavailable," says Dr. Gordon Weir, of Harvard University's Joslin Diabetes Center in Boston.

Weir, who is recruiting patients for his own study of the Edmonton procedure, says he expected the transplants to meet with less-than-universal success. "I'm not surprised that some of them would have failed, and I assume more will fail. I never thought it would be a lifetime of normal blood sugars."

Several other research centers, including the University of Miami, the University of Minnesota and institutes in Europe, are performing islet cell transplants using procedures similar to the Edmonton Protocol. While these trials are important in the effort to cure diabetes, Deb Butterfield, executive director of the Insulin Free World Foundation in

St. Louis, says the more significant breakthrough will come when scientists can graft islets without needing an entire pancreas to gather the cells.

Roughly 5,000 pancreases a year are available for transplant in the United States, and of those only about 1,500 of the operations are performed, Butterfield says. Current islet cell transplants require at least one if not two pancreases per patient, she says, where ideally the situation would be two or three patients per organ.

Still, with about 1.5 million Type 1 diabetics in the United States alone—compared with 15 million with Type 2 (non-insulin-dependent) diabetes—the number of donor pancreases will never meet the demand for them.

"We have to move toward cell therapies," such as stem cell manipulation or cloning, says Butterfield.

Coping with Immune-Suppressing Drugs

Another important breakthrough will be finding ways to obviate immune-suppressing drugs that keep the body from rejecting transplanted tissue, Butterfield says. Researchers in Miami are now following a patient who received a bone marrow transplant in addition to islet cells as a way to prime his immune system to accept the donor tissue.

But bone marrow transplants, which are themselves traumatic, may not be necessary, says Ryan, who cites recent animal studies showing that it may be possible to wean graft recipients off drugs yet maintain the donor cells. "There's hope," Ryan says. "But it's very early days yet."

Teskey, who keeps in touch with his fellow transplant recipients, admits that he's among the fortunate ones. "For me it has gone amazingly well," says Teskey. "I'm now two years out from the transplants and have been off insulin completely for that entire time."

Not only that, but he has been spared the worst of the immune-suppressing regimen, though he does have to watch for surges in his blood pressure and in the beginning he was plagued by painful mouth sores. "Those minor difficulties are really very insignificant in comparison with the positive change in my life," he adds.

Dale Camp, another transplant recipient, hasn't been so lucky. The grafts, placed in May and June of 1999, helped stabilize Camp's blood sugar. But the immune-quelling drugs have been murder. "The islets have done reasonably well, but the side effects have been quite poor," Camp says. "I've had a pretty rough time."

Diarrhea and trouble absorbing food have dropped his weight from 150 pounds to as low as 115 pounds, though lately it has come up a bit. Apparently unrelated to the drugs, his white blood cell count plunged to "next to nothing."

"They've given me quite a ride," Camp says of the medications, in his case tacrolimus and Rapamune. Still, Camp, who was diagnosed with diabetes in 1949 at the age of 2, doesn't feel he made a mistake enrolling in the trial. "I was in a push-and-shove-type situation. I was hypo-unaware and had severe insulin reactions many times a day or week. It was just a matter of time before I didn't wake up from one." Keeping his insulin in line "is not only good for me, it's good for my wife and everyone around me as well," Camp says.

Yet Camp, who lives in Falun, Alberta, is philosophical about the tradeoff, and says it was a risk he was willing to take. "If you wish to keep your transplant, you have to maintain some sort of a level of immune suppression, and you're going to be with it the rest of your life. We're a new technology here, and everybody's learning and everybody's very individual," he adds. "For some people it works and for some people it might not. That's sort of the luck of the draw."

BATTLING DIABETIC EYE DISEASE

Jim Brabenec and Lance Cheung

After twenty-one years in the U.S. Air Force, Tech. Sgt. Miguel DeLeon Jr. lost his battle against diabetic eye disease and was forced to retire from the only career he ever wanted. But DeLeon did not give up without a fight, Jim Brabenec and Lance Cheung write in the following selection. DeLeon used his creativity to accommodate his loss of vision, the authors report. In some situations, they observe, DeLeon would have people describe problems he would then visualize and solve, and in others, family members and friends would serve as his eyes. According to the authors, these efforts became an inspiration to those who served on his team in the 9th Transportation Squadron. Although DeLeon's battle against the complications of diabetes is far from over, the authors relate that he and his family will continue the fight. Tech. Sgts. Brabenec and Cheung write for the *Airman*, a publication of the U.S. Air Force, Air Force News Agency.

Some people say they know their jobs so well that they can do them with their eyes closed.

Retired Tech. Sgt. Miguel DeLeon Jr. believed he could do that. But he learned differently.

He had to use a magnifying glass to read, set up golfball-sized icons on his computer just to see them, and write with magic markers so he could see the words easier.

Unfortunately, diabetes dealt this warrior a severe blow—nearly robbing him of his sight. And because he had uncorrectable vision and was legally blind, he was medically retired from the Air Force in February 2001, after 21 years of service.

"My vision just wasn't there," he said. "And even though I didn't want to go, I accepted it."

DeLeon spent his last 10 years in the Air Force fighting the disease. He changed his diet, watched his weight and studied the enemy. To no avail.

"Some people would have just given up," said Matt, DeLeon's 13-

Excerpted from "DeLeon vs. Diabetes," by Jim Brabenec and Lance Cheung, *Airman*, April 2001.

year-old son, as he helped his father test his blood sugar level. "But my dad's still doing great things. I'm proud of him."

Accommodating a Loss of Vision

Care, concern and a large dose of creativity have been DeLeon's approach to life and his mission. As the 9th Transportation Squadron's superintendent of combat readiness at Beale Air Force Base, Calif., the job he held before retiring, he led trainers who taught units how to deploy their people and equipment.

"I pride myself on giving 200 percent of myself, but with my bad eyes I can only give 100 percent," DeLeon said. He realized it was "time to move on. Even though I tried to do the things I used to, I had difficulty. My vision isn't there."

That wasn't easy for a hard-charger like DeLeon to admit. Described as "an extraordinary troubleshooter with a wealth of knowledge" by his former boss Maj. Monte Murphy, 9th Transportation Squadron commander, things began to unravel for him near the end of his career.

His eyesight got so bad that if someone had a problem, DeLeon had to ask him to describe it. From that he would form a picture and try to solve it.

Inside DeLeon's office, things looked much the same as any other Air Force member's at first glance. On the walls, photographs of austere locations proved he never turned down the chance to deploy. A large computer monitor dominated his desk space. In fact everything dealing with the written language was large.

This growth of letters and numbers wasn't for fun; it was out of necessity.

To look at something, he used peripheral vision because his central vision is permanently blurred. Consequently, when he talked to people, he appeared to be scanning around them rather than looking directly at them.

While he altered his physical workspace to meet his needs, DeLeon also relied on those close to him to help meet many of the other demands of life.

"My family and co-workers were tremendously supportive, and they helped me feel valuable," DeLeon said. They helped him with rides to work or identifying things he couldn't quite focus on. Of his former unit, he said it was a "great team, and I'm very thankful for them."

One of those former team members said it's she who is thankful.

"I've learned so much more than just the job from Sergeant DeLeon," said 2nd Lt. Kate Nenni, the squadron's combat readiness flight commander.

DeLeon served as Nenni's technical mentor, but she said just as importantly, his battle with his disease taught her something about living her own life.

"I have to take care of myself when I'm young," she said. "Having realized this through his example, I try to live life to the fullest and thank God for the gifts I've been given. Because in a flash it can all change."

A Life Changed

And, oh, how life has changed for DeLeon. It's the subtle things he laments most.

"If I'm telling a joke to my son, I can't tell his reaction because I can't see the smile on his face," he said.

And ending his Air Force career is still difficult for him.

"The Air Force is all I ever wanted [to do]," he said. Now he has to reinvent himself for a life without vision.

DeLeon's high blood sugar levels weakened the delicate blood vessels of his eyes' retinas. The weakest of these vessels swell and interfere with the optic nerves. The progressive swelling will disconnect the light sensors of his eyes from the optic nerves, leaving him completely blind. Eventually there will be life-threatening complications, but the DeLeon family is resolved to do whatever it takes to battle this disease and live life to the fullest.

DeLeon is attending vocational rehabilitation at a veteran's hospital and the Lighthouse for the Blind. He's pursuing an education in teaching to work with high school age kids and hopes to be a touring speaker for hospital diabetic teaching programs while continuing his fight in Newport News, Va.

For a warrior like DeLeon, it's obvious being legally blind hasn't affected his focus.

"THROUGH THE EYES OF THE EAGLE": A NATIVE AMERICAN VISION

Georgia Perez

Georgia Perez is a Native American from the Pueblo of Nambe and coordinator of the University of New Mexico Native American Diabetes Project (NADP). Perez wrote the following story in an effort to make the message of the NADP relevant to Native Americans by incorporating elements of Native American culture. In this selection, the Eagle, a respected Native American symbol, tells the story of a people who were once active and nourished by Mother Earth. The Eagle is troubled, however, by changes that have made the people sick with "Too Much Sugar in the Blood." But the Eagle has a vision that the people become healthy and strong when they learn the wisdom of leading a healthier lifestyle.

The University of New Mexico Native American Diabetes Project (NADP) "Strong in Body & Spirit!" curriculum represents a unique approach to diabetes education among Native Americans. Unlike other diabetes education programs, NADP interweaves its health message with the traditions and stories that have been—and continue to be—an essential aspect of the Native American culture.

"Through the Eyes of the Eagle" is one example of how the NADP curriculum makes its diabetes messages relevant to its audience.

Georgia Perez, from the Pueblo of Nambe, who wrote the story—which came to her in a dream—adds, "Because the eagle is a religious and highly respected symbolic figure within our culture, I felt that this story, and the eagle, would be valuable additions to our project."

"Through the Eyes of the Eagle"

This is the land of my Native People. As I soar high above through the clouds, I see the beauty Mother Earth provides for my people, from the high peaks of the mountaintops where the rivers begin, to the valleys below where the waters run through.

I see Brother Sun as he greets each day with his morning light, and I see him fade to make room for Sister Moon.

As each day comes, the bear, the cougar, the deer, and I see the children, so pretty with a tan of golden brown, playing and running in their communities. The men, with their legs so strong, keep up with the antelope as they run. The women, so beautiful as they work, make their families healthy and strong.

I remember when running was a way of life for everyone and so was living off Mother Earth with what she provided. Times were hard but the Native People all worked together and shared in their labors and good fortunes through many feasts and celebrations. People came from far and near to join them in giving thanks to the Great Spirit for all that they were given and for a long and healthy life.

Brother Sun and Sister Moon have come and gone many times as I continue to fly over the land of my Native People. As each passing day goes by, I have seen many changes, some good and some bad. Mother Earth is still the same, for she continues to provide nourishment for all living things, large and small. And she provides beauty for all to see and enjoy.

But now I feel troubled and sad that I no longer see my Native people enjoying what Mother Earth has for them. With changing times, their labors are still hard but I see them not as strong as they could be. Modern days have brought about many changes so that my people no longer run like the antelope.

Children seldom play but watch what they call television. My people are getting sick by threes and fours with this thing called "Too Much Sugar in the Blood."

My Native People of golden brown no longer have the strength of their ancestors. As I soar through the clouds, I now see my people no longer active.

They suffer from lost vision and strength. Their feet, that once carried them over the lands of their birth, suffer great pain. Some of my people of golden brown now use wheels to get around, and others need machines to keep their bodies clean.

Oh, what a sad vision that my eyes now see. If only there was some way to give my people of golden brown my courage and strength to turn this around.

As I come to rest on my mountaintop, I close my eyes, tired from what I have seen, and begin to see another vision of how it can be to bring back the strength, courage, and long life to my people of golden brown.

My Native People are getting out and around. Slowly they come out, by ones and twos, to work and enjoy the riches and beauty that Mother Earth gives. They are walking and beginning to run and slowly get stronger as their sugars come down. As others see them getting stronger, they too want the same, so they join in until all are doing the same. They once again talk and share their ideas of what they can do to continue to grow healthier too.

They begin slowly by making one change, then two, to eat less sugar and less fat things too. As they grow stronger and continue to make these changes, they come to know that they are healthier, not only in body but in mind and spirit, too, as they now can control this thing called "Too Much Sugar in the Blood."

Their children and grandchildren now know what they can do to grow and become stronger and healthier, too. By learning and through examples taught by their parents and grandparents, they have obtained the wisdom of knowing what they need to do to keep their sugars down and have a healthier lifestyle.

As a new day approaches with Brother Sun bringing his light, I no longer feel troubled, for I know they will learn what they can do to make my vision at rest all come to pass.

My Native People of golden brown will once again be healthy and strong as they make the necessary changes to turn things around and once again will be Strong in Body and Spirit!

GLOSSARY

albumin: A protein found in blood plasma and urine, which can be a sign of kidney disease.

atherosclerosis: The buildup of cholesterol and other fat deposits, known as plaque, on the inner layer of an artery.

beta cells: Cells that make insulin, found in areas of the pancreas called the islets of Langerhans.

blood glucose: The main sugar that the body makes from food; cells cannot use glucose without the help of insulin.

cardiovascular disease: A disease of the heart or blood vessels.

diabetes mellitus: A disorder that prevents the body from converting digested food into the energy needed for daily activities.

gestational diabetes: A form of diabetes that begins during pregnancy in women who were not known to have diabetes before and usually disappears following delivery.

glucose: A sugar in the blood, and a source of energy for the body.

glucose tolerance test: A blood test used to diagnose diabetes, including gestational diabetes.

hemoglobin A1c: A test that indicates how much glucose has been sticking to part of the hemoglobin during the past three to four months.

high-density lipoprotein (HDL) cholesterol: Known as the "good cholesterol," HDL is believed to carry cholesterol to the liver for removal from the body.

hyperglycemia: A condition that occurs in people with diabetes when their blood glucose levels are too high.

hypoglycemia: A condition in which the blood sugar is lower than normal.

immunosuppression drugs: Drugs that impair the body's ability to fight infection or recognize foreign substances that enter the body; a person receiving a transplant is given these drugs to stop the body from rejecting the new organ or tissue.

impaired glucose tolerance (IGT): A condition in which blood sugar levels are higher than normal but are not high enough to be classified as diabetes; a risk factor for type 2 diabetes.

insulin: A hormone manufactured by the pancreas that helps glucose leave the blood and enter the muscles and other tissues of the body.

insulin-dependent diabetes: Also known as type 1 diabetes, a condition in which the pancreas makes so little insulin that the body cannot use blood glucose as energy; it must be controlled with daily insulin injections.

insulin resistance: Partial blocking of the effect of insulin.

ketoacidosis: High blood glucose, often caused by illness or taking too little insulin.

ketone: Breakdown product of fat that accumulates in the blood as a result of inadequate insulin or inadequate calorie intake.

low-density lipoprotein (LDL) cholesterol: Known as the "bad cholesterol," LDL in high levels can deposit on the walls of the blood vessel and can cause formation of plaques.

macrosomia: Term meaning "large body" that refers to a baby that is considered larger than normal, a condition that occurs when the mother's blood sugar levels have been higher than normal during the pregnancy; a preventable complication of gestational diabetes.

nephropathy: Diabetic kidney disease.

neuropathy: Diabetic nerve damage.

non-insulin-dependent diabetes: Also known as type 2 diabetes, a condition in which the body either makes too little insulin or cannot use the insulin it makes to use blood glucose as energy; it can often be controlled through meal plans, physical activity plans, and diabetes pills or insulin.

pancreas: The long gland that lies behind the stomach that manufactures insulin and digestive enzymes.

retinopathy: Diabetic eye disease.

self-monitoring blood glucose: A method for people with diabetes to find out how much glucose is in their blood.

triglycerides: A type of fat in the blood that increases after a person eats.

ORGANIZATIONS TO CONTACT

The editors have compiled the following list of organizations concerned with the issues presented in this book. Descriptions are derived from materials provided by the organizations. All have publications or information available for interested readers. The list was compiled on the date of publication of the present volume; the information provided here may change. Be aware that many organizations take several weeks or longer to respond to inquiries, so allow as much time as possible.

American Association of Diabetes Educators (AADE)
100 West Monroe, 4th Floor, Chicago, IL 60603
(312) 424-2426 • fax: (312) 424-2427
e-mail: aade@aadenet.org • website: www.aadenet.org

AADE is a multidisciplinary organization representing over 10,000 health-care professionals whose goal is to advance the role of the diabetes educator and improve the quality of diabetes education and care. The association publishes the latest diabetes education research along with valuable teaching tools and techniques, including *A Core Curriculum for Diabetes Education*, a comprehensive diabetes education resource; the *Diabetes Educator*, a bimonthly journal for the diabetes health-care team; and the *AADE News*. On its website, the association provides a search engine to locate local diabetes educators, access to its research database, and links to related sites.

American Diabetes Association (ADA)
National Service Center
1701 North Beauregard St., Alexandria, VA 22311
(703) 549-1500 or (800) 232-3472 • fax: (703) 549-6996
e-mail: customerservice@diabetes.org • website: www.diabetes.org

The ADA is a nonprofit health organization providing diabetes research, information, and advocacy. The mission of the organization is to prevent and cure diabetes and to improve the lives of all people affected by diabetes. To fulfill this mission, the ADA funds research, publishes scientific findings, and provides information and other services to people with diabetes, their families, health-care professionals, and the public. The association is also actively involved in advocating for scientific research and for the rights of people with diabetes. The ADA publishes many books and resources for health professionals and people with diabetes, including *Diabetes Forecast*, a monthly magazine for people with diabetes; and *Clinical Diabetes, Diabetes, Diabetes Care* and *Diabetes Spectrum*, for health-care professionals. On its website, the ADA provides news and information on type 1 and type 2 diabetes, a search engine to obtain local information, and access to some of its journal articles.

Centers for Disease Control and Prevention (CDC)
National Center for Chronic Disease Prevention and Health Promotion
Division of Diabetes Translation
Mail Stop K-10
4770 Buford Highway NE, Atlanta, GA 30341-3717
(800) CDC-DIAB • fax: (301) 562-1050
e-mail: diabetes@cdc.gov • website: www.cdc.gov/diabetes

The mission of the diabetes division of the CDC is to reduce the burden of diabetes in the United States by planning, conducting, coordinating, and evaluating federal efforts to translate promising results of diabetes research into widespread clinical and public health practice. The CDC distributes several publications, including a guide for people with diabetes, a diabetes surveillance report, and the eight-page *National Diabetes Fact Sheet: National Estimates and General Information on Diabetes in the United States*. On its diabetes website, the CDC provides access to fact sheets, statistics, publications, and information about state diabetes control programs.

Children with Diabetes Foundation
2525 Arapahoe Ave., Suite E4, Boulder, CO 80302
e-mail: info@CWDFoundation.org • website: www.cwdfoundation.org

The Children with Diabetes Foundation was founded by a group, mostly parents of children with diabetes, who are committed to finding a cure for type 1 diabetes. The goal of the foundation is to assist people living with diabetes and support the work of scientists and physicians throughout the world searching for a cure. On its website, the foundation provides access to an online community, research updates, and other diabetes news.

Diabetes Exercise and Sports Association (DESA)
PO Box 1935, Litchfield Park, AZ 85340
(623) 535-4593 or (800) 898-4322 • fax: (623) 535-4741
e-mail: desa@diabetes-exercise.org • website: www.diabetes-exercise.org

DESA exists to enhance the quality of life for people with diabetes through exercise and physical fitness. Its activities include creating recreational, sport, and athletic activities; providing a forum for support, sharing, and exchange of ideas and experiences; and educating health professionals who work with active individuals with diabetes. DESA publishes a quarterly newsletter, the *Challenge*, which includes technology updates and accounts of diabetic athletes, their activities, and their achievements.

Insulin-Free World Foundation
677 Craig Rd., Suite 105, St. Louis, MO 63141-7115
(314) 991-8004 • fax: (314) 991-2276
e-mail: info@insulinfree.org • website: www.insulin-free.org

Founded in 1996 to facilitate the exchange of information in the diabetes community, the Insulin-Free World Foundation corresponds with diabetes researchers and clinicians at prominent academic institutions, gathering research articles, facts and statistics, scientific abstracts, human-interest stories, and other information about advances in insulin-free treatments and cures for diabetes. The foundation also hosts an online directory of pancreas and islet transplant specialists and initiates and hosts campaigns to amplify the public outcry against diabetes to shift public attention from managing to curing diabetes. The foundation distributes information on its website and in its quarterly magazine, *Insulin-Free TIMES*, which integrates information about advances toward curing diabetes with current social, political, and economic issues affecting the diabetic community.

Joslin Diabetes Center
One Joslin Pl., Boston, MA 02215
(617) 732-2400 • website: www.joslin.harvard.edu

The Joslin Diabetes Center offers inpatient and outpatient treatment, education, and other support services to adults and children with diabetes; provides professional medical education; sponsors camps for children with diabetes; and supports research to improve treatment and find a cure for diabetes and its complications. The center is affiliated with Harvard Medical School and a number of hospitals in the Boston area and operates affiliated clinics in several states. The Joslin Diabetes Center is one of six diabetes endocrinology research centers supported by the National Institute of Diabetes and Digestive and Kidney Diseases. The center publishes educational materials for patients and professionals, some of which are available on its website, including manuals, nutrition guides, materials for children with diabetes, films, and the quarterly *Joslin Magazine.*

Juvenile Diabetes Research Foundation International (JDRF)
120 Wall St., 19th Floor, New York, NY 10005
(800) 533-2873 or (212) 785-9500 • fax: (212) 785-9595
e-mail: infor@jdf.org • website: www.jdf.org

JDRF was founded in 1970 by the parents of children with juvenile diabetes, a disease that strikes children suddenly, makes them insulin dependent for life, and carries the constant threat of devastating complications. The foundation is an international, nonprofit, voluntary health agency that supports and funds research to find a cure for diabetes and its complications. JDRF has three major goals: restoring normal blood sugar, preventing and reversing diabetes-related complications, and preventing diabetes and its recurrence. The foundation publishes the quarterly journal *Countdown* and a series of patient education brochures about type 1 and type 2 diabetes. On its website, the foundation provides news about its efforts, information about diabetes, and access to excerpts from its publications.

National Diabetes Alliance
4050 N. Maiden Dr., Baton Rouge, LA 70809
(225) 927-0317 • fax: (225) 928-0540
e-mail: mail@diabetesalliance.org • website:http://diabetesalliance.org

The mission of the alliance is to assist independent and allied diabetes organizations to improve the physical and social well-being of persons with diabetes. It is not a centralized agency but coordinates a project-by-project partnership of independent diabetes organizations throughout America, providing local organizations with access to unified national diabetes projects while maintaining their independent local governance. The alliance publishes an online magazine, *Diabetes America,* which brings visitors the latest news and articles pertaining to diabetes, including live seminars.

National Institutes of Health (NIH)
National Institute of Diabetes and Digestive and Kidney Diseases (NIDDK)
National Diabetes Information Clearinghouse (NDIC)
1 Information Way, Bethesda, MD 20892-3560
fax: (301) 907-8906
e-mail: nidic@infor.niddk.nih.gov
website: www.niddk.nih.gov/health/diabetes/diabetes.htm

The NDIC is a service of the NIDDK, the government's lead agency for diabetes research. NIDDK operates three information clearinghouses and funds six diabetes research and training centers and eight diabetes endocrinology research centers. Established in 1978, the NDIC serves as a diabetes information, education, and referral resource for people with diabetes, their families, health-care professionals, and the public. The NDIC publishes a semiannual newsletter, *Diabetes Dateline,* and website visitors may conduct literature searches on a myriad of subjects related to diabetes.

BIBLIOGRAPHY

Books

American Diabetes Association	*American Diabetes Association Complete Guide to Diabetes: The Ultimate Home Diabetes Reference.* 2nd ed. Alexandria, VA: American Diabetes Association, 1999.
Sheri R. Colberg	*The Diabetic Athlete.* Champaign, IL: Human Kinetics, 2001.
Denis Daneman, Marcia Frank, and Kusiel Perlman	*When a Child Has Diabetes.* Buffalo, NY: Firefly Books, 1999.
Eve Gehling	*The Family and Friends' Guide to Diabetes: Everything You Need to Know.* New York: Wiley, 2000.
Diana W. Guthrie	*Alternative and Complementary Diabetes Care: How to Combine Natural and Traditional Therapies.* New York: Wiley, 2000.
Debra Haire-Joshu, ed.	*Management of Diabetes Mellitus: Perspective of Care Across the Life Span.* St. Louis: Mosby-Year Book, 1996.
Linda O'Neill	*Having Diabetes.* Vero Beach, FL: Rourke Press, 2001.
Victoria Peurrung	*Living with Juvenile Diabetes: A Practical Guide for Parents and Caregivers.* New York: Hatherleigh Press, 2001.
Robert H. Phillips	*Coping with Diabetes: Sound, Compassionate Advice to Alleviate the Challenges of Type I and Type II Diabetes.* Garden City, NY: Avery, 2000.
Laurinda M. Poirer and Katharine M. Coburn	*Women and Diabetes: Staying Healthy in Body, Mind, and Spirit.* Alexandria, VA: American Diabetes Association, 2000.
Simeon I. Taylor, ed.	*Current Review of Diabetes.* Philadelphia: Current Medicine, 1999.
Douglas Wetherill and Dean J. Kereiakes	*Diabetes: What You Should Know.* Cincinnati: Betterway Books, 2000.
Julian Whitaker	*Reversing Diabetes.* New York: Warner Books, 2001.

Periodicals

Jerry Adler et al.	"An American Epidemic," *Newsweek*, September 4, 2000.
Edwin W. Brown	"Diabetes: Still a Deadly Disease," *Medical Update*, November 1997. Available from the American Foundation for Preventive Medicine, 1102 Stadium Dr., Indianapolis, IN 46202.
Neelima V. Chu and Steven V. Edelman	"Diabetes and Erectile Dysfunction," *Clinical Diabetes*, Winter 2001. Available from the American Diabetes Association, 1701 N. Beauregard St., Alexandria, VA 22311.

Charles M. Clark Jr.   "The National Diabetes Education Program: Changing the Way Diabetes Is Treated," *Diabetes Care*, April 2001. Available from the American Diabetes Association, 1701 N. Beauregard St., Alexandria, VA 22311.

Wayne L. Clark   "Pumped Up, but Is It for Everyone?" *Countdown*, Fall 1997. Available from the Juvenile Diabetes Foundation, 120 Wall St., New York, NY 10005-4001.

Terri D'Arrigo   "All in the Family: Kidney Disease and Type 1," *Diabetes Forecast*, April 1999. Available from the American Diabetes Association, 1701 N. Beauregard St., Alexandria, VA 22311.

Nancy Walsh D'Epiro and Michelle Johnson   "Reducing the Burden of Diabetes and CVD," *Patient Care*, May 15, 2000. Available from Five Paragon Dr., Montvale, NJ 07645-1742.

Steven V. Edelman   "Prevention, Early Detection, and Aggressive Management of Diabetic Kidney Disease," *Clinical Diabetes*, 1998.

Michael Fumento   "Vietnam Flashback: Diabetes–Agent Orange Connection," *Reason*, July 2000.

James R. Gavin III   "Diabetes: African American Program," *Ebony*, March 1999.

David Goetzl   "Rate of Diabetes in Ethnic Groups Sparks Outreach," *Advertising Age*, November 20, 2000. Available from Reprint Management Services, (717) 399-1900.

Sheldon H. Gottlieb   "'K-Ration': Diabetes and Cardiovascular Risk," *Diabetes Forecast*, February 2002.

Sari Harrar and Paula Rasich   "Beat Diabetes Before It Starts," *Prevention*, November 2001.

Irl B. Hirsch   "The Heart of Diabetes," *Clinical Diabetes*, Fall 2000.

Bonnie Liebman   "How to Cut Your Risk of Diabetes," *Nutrition Action Healthletter*, May 2001. Available from 1875 Connecticut Ave. NW, Suite 300, Washington, DC 20009.

Hugh McDevitt   "Closing In on Type 1 Diabetes," *New England Journal of Medicine*, October 4, 2001. Available from the Massachusetts Medical Society, 860 Winter St., Waltham, MA 02451-1413.

Meng Hee Tan   "Diabetes and Coronary Heart Disease," *Diabetes Spectrum*, Spring 1999. Available from the American Diabetes Association, 1701 N. Beauregard St., Alexandria, VA 22311.

Sharon Scott Morey   "AHA Examines Cardiovascular Problems in Diabetes," *American Family Physician*, January 15, 2000. Available from 11400 Tomakawk Creek Pkwy., Leawood, KS 66211-2672.

Laurinda
Poirier-Soloman

"Eating Disorders and Diabetes," *Diabetes Forecast,*
November 2001.

Laurinda
Poirier-Soloman

"Taking It to Heart," *Diabetes Forecast,* February 2001.

Raymond L. Reynolds

"Reemergence of Insulin Pump Therapy in the 1990s,"
Southern Medical Journal, December 2000. Available
from the Southern Medical Association, SMJ, PO Box
190088, Birmingham, AL 35219-0088.

R. Paul Robertson

"Successful Islet Transplantation for Patients with
Diabetes: Fact or Fantasy?" *New England Journal of
Medicine,* July 27, 2000.

Arlan L. Rosenbloom

"Not 'Adults-Only' Anymore," *Diabetes Forecast,*
March 2001.

Joannie M. Schrof

"The Silent Killer," *U.S. News & World Report,* April 12,
1999.

Stacey Schultz

"Living with Diabetes: A Cure Could Be on the Way,"
U.S. News & World Report, August 7, 2000.

Shawn Shepherd

"Diabetes Cost on the Rise," *Business Press,* January 22,
1999. Available from 3700 Inland Empire Blvd., Suite
450, Ontario, CA 91764.

P.A. Tataranni and
C. Bogardus

"Changing Habits to Delay Diabetes," *New England
Journal of Medicine,* May 3, 2001.

Mike Terry

"Discovering Diabetes," *Essence,* January 1999.

INDEX

reactions to, 53
resistance, 8, 15, 22, 32, 58, 101,
  122, 124
  adolescence and, 59
  obesity and, 59, 75–76, 106
  thrifty genotype and, 59, 64
Insulin Free World Foundation, 154
International Diabetes Federation
  (IDF), 21
International Diabetes Institute, 21
International Histocompatibility
  Working Group, 87
International Islet Transplant
  Registry, 119
International Type 1 Diabetes
  Genetics Consortium, 87

Juneja, Rattan, 57
Juvenile Diabetes Foundation, 11, 139
Juvenile Diabetes Foundation
  International (JDF), 18, 39, 45
  Center for Complications of
    Diabetes, 40–42, 45
Juvenile Diabetes Research
  Foundation International (JDRF),
  87, 88, 90–91

King, Hilary, 63
Knowler, Bill, 74, 76–77
Kolata, Gina, 78
Kong, Waine, 33

Leeuwenburg, Jay, 137–39

Marcus, Adam, 153
McCance, D.R., 65
McCarren, Marie, 147
McDonough, John, 39–41, 45
Medicare, 117
Mertz, W., 128
Michalek, Joel E., 78–80
Micro-Hope studies, 25
Morgan, Peggy, 135

Nathan, David, 94–95
National Institute of Allergy and
  Infectious Diseases (NIAID), 87–90
National Institute of Arthritis and
  Musculoskeletal and Skin Diseases
  (NIAMS), 89
National Institute of Child Health
  and Human Development
  (NICHD), 88–89, 91
National Institute of Dental and
  Craniofacial Research (NIDCR), 89

National Institute of Diabetes and
  Digestive and Kidney Diseases
  (NIDDKD), 9, 13
  Diabetes Prevention Program
    (DPP), 20, 61, 93–95, 150–51
  Diabetes Prevention Trial—Type 1,
    19
  genetics research, 87–88
  Pima Indian study, 73–77
  Transplantation and
    Autoimmunity Branch, 89
  type 1 research, 87–92
National Institute of Environmental
  Health Sciences (NIEHS), 88
National Institute of Neurological
  Disorders and Stroke (NINDS), 91
National Institute of Nursing
  Research, 91
National Institutes of Health (NIH)
  research by, 18, 87
  Immune Tolerance Network
    (ITN), 89, 90
  increase in type 2 diabetes, 8–9
  Office of Research on Women's
    Health (ORWH), 89
Native Americans
  Diabetes Prevention Program, 20,
    94, 151
  education and, 160–62
  high risk for diabetes, 8, 15–16,
    23–24, 83, 148
  Pima Indians, 16, 58, 65, 73–77
  thrifty genotype, 58–59, 65, 70–71
Neel, James, 58, 63–66
niacin, 129–30
niacinamide, 129–30

obesity
  as cause of diabetes, 8–9, 14–15,
    22–25, 59, 67–72, 75–77, 82–85,
    100–101, 148
  insulin resistance and, 59, 75–76,
    106
  thrifty genotype and, 58–59, 64
Ofili, Elizabeth, 32
Opsal, Christen, 143
oral glucose tolerance test (OGTT),
  15, 95

Parkinson's disease, 45
Peragallo-Dittko, Virginia, 111
Perez, Georgia, 160
Perry, Patrick, 57
Pianoforte, Kerry, 137
Pima Indians, 16, 58, 65, 73–77